CW00691077

HOW TO QUIT SMOKING

A Complete Guide on How to Stop Smoking,
Permanently

Derek Sullivan

UP

URANUS
PUBLISHING

Uranus Publishing

Contents

INTRODUCTION

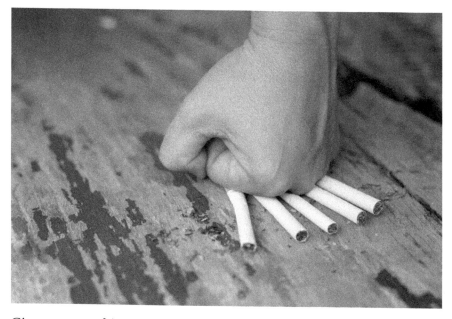

Cigarette smoking is one of the biggest preventable causes of mortality in the United States, yet quitting can be difficult.

Many people believe that witnessing gains in health and well-being will take a long time, yet the timescale for seeing meaningful benefits is shorter than most people anticipate.

Here are some crucial points for quitting smoking. More information and supporting evidence can be found in the main article.

- Quitting smoking entails breaking the cycle of addiction and reprogramming the brain to no longer need nicotine.
- To be successful, smokers who wish to stop must have a strategy to deal with cravings and triggers.
- The benefits of quitting smoking can be felt as soon as one hour after the last cigarette is smoked.
- The sooner a smoker quits, the sooner they will minimize their risk of cancer, heart disease, and other smoking-related diseases.

Now think about your situation.

You're considering stopping smoking. Do you understand why you want to quit? Do you wish to improve your health? Do you want to save money? How do you keep your family safe? Why are there so many reasons?

If you're not sure, consider the following:

- What is it about smoking that I dislike?
- When I smoke, what do I miss out on?
- What is the impact of smoking on my health?
- What will become of my family and me if I continue to smoke?
- When I quit, how will my life improve?

Remind yourself of your reasons for quitting every day once you've identified them. It has the potential to motivate you to quit Smoking for good.

- Do you want to be, look, and feel better?

Here are a few additional reasons to think about it.

Cancer, heart attacks, heart disease, stroke, cataracts, and other ailments will be less likely to strike me.

I'll be less likely to develop colds or the flu, and if I do, I'll be able to recover faster.

I could breathe more easily and cough less.

My blood pressure is going to drop.

My skin will be better, and I will appear younger.

There will be no stains on my teeth or fingernails.

Quitting Smoking will improve your health and make you feel better. There are, however, other reasons to quit that you may not have considered.

- Want to live a healthy lifestyle?
I'll be able to spend more money.

I can catch up on work or pursue my favorite hobby.

I won't have to worry about when I'll be able to smoke again or where I'll be able to smoke.

My cuisine will be more flavorful.

My garments will have a more pleasant odor.

My car, house, and children will not smell like a cigarette.

I'll be able to smell things like food, flowers, and other things more clearly.

- Want to have a better family life?

I'll set a good example for my children by quitting; it takes a lot of courage to do so.

My loved ones, including my friends, family, coworkers, and others, will be proud of me.

I will safeguard my friends and family from second-hand smoke risks.

My children will be in better health.

I'll have more energy to spend with my friends and family doing the activities I enjoy.

I'm going to get healthy, so I can be there for my family's important occasions.

I wrote this book to help people solve their smoking problems and improve their lives. Right now, it may seem not very easy, but many others before you have succeeded, and with the correct information, you will too.

It's time to get to work!

Chapter One

EFFECTS OF SMOKING ON YOUR LIFE

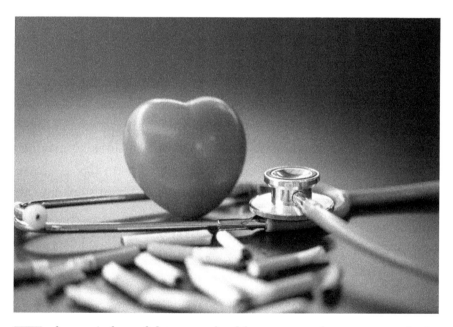

Tobacco is harmful to your health no matter how you smoke it. There are no safe compounds in cigarette products, from acetone and tar to nicotine and carbon monoxide. The things you inhale have an impact on more than simply your lungs. They have the potential to harm your entire body.

Smoking can cause a number of long-term health problems as well as long-term consequences on your bodily systems. While smoking increases your risk of some issues over time, some of the physical impacts are seen right away.

Tobacco smoke is extremely hazardous to one's health. There is no such thing as a safe way to smoke. You won't be able to escape the health dangers by substituting a cigar, pipe, or hookah for your cigarette.

About 600 components are contained in cigarettes, many of which are also found in cigars and hookahs. According to the American Lung Association, they produce over 7,000 toxins when these substances burn. Many of the compounds are toxic, and at least 69 have been related to cancer.

In the United States, smokers have a threefold higher mortality rate than non-smokers. According to the Centers for Disease Control and Prevention (CDC), smoking is the most common "preventable cause of death" in the United States. While the effects of smoking may not be noticeable right away, the complications and harm that it causes might persist for years. The good news is that stopping smoking can reverse many negative consequences.

Central nervous system

Nicotine, a mood-altering chemical, is one of the constituents of tobacco. Nicotine reaches your brain in seconds and gives you a temporary energy boost. However, as the effect wears off, you become tired and hungry for more. Nicotine is incredibly addictive, which is why quitting smoking is so tough.

Nicotine withdrawal can decrease cognitive performance and leave you feeling anxious, irritable, and sad. Withdrawal might also lead to headaches and insomnia.

Respiratory system

Inhaling smoke exposes your lungs to toxins that can harm them. This injury causes a slew of issues over time. Along with an increased risk of infection, smokers are more likely to develop chronic nonreversible lung diseases such as:

- The destruction of the air sacs in your lungs is known as emphysema.
- Chronic bronchitis is long-term inflammation of the lining of the lungs' breathing tubes.
- A category of lung disorders is known as a chronic obstructive pulmonary disease (COPD).
- lung cancer

As your lungs and airways heal, withdrawal from tobacco products might cause temporary congestion and respiratory discomfort. Mucus production spikes shortly after quitting smoking, indicating that your respiratory system is recuperating.

Coughing, wheezing, and asthma attacks are more common in children whose parents smoke than in children whose parents do not smoke. They're also more likely to get pneumonia or bronchitis.

Cardiovascular system

Smoking harms your cardiovascular system as a whole. Nicotine causes blood arteries to constrict, restricting blood flow. Peripheral artery disease can develop over time due to continuous constriction and damage to the blood arteries.

Smoking also causes blood clots, elevates blood pressure, and weakens blood vessel walls. This increases your chance of a stroke when taken together.

If you've already had heart bypass surgery, a heart attack, or a stent implanted in a blood vessel, you're at a higher risk of deteriorating heart disease.

Smoking has an impact not only on your cardiovascular health but also on the health of individuals who do not smoke. Nonsmokers are at the same risk as smokers when they are exposed to secondhand smoke. Stroke, heart attack, and heart disease are all risks.

Integumentary system

Skin alterations are one of the more visible indications of smoking. Tobacco smoke contains substances that alter the structure of your skin. According to a new study, smoking significantly increases the risk of squamous cell carcinoma (skin cancer).

The effects of smoking can be felt on your fingernails and toenails. Fungal nail infections are more likely if you smoke.

Nicotine affects hair as well. According to an older study, it causes hair loss, baldness, and graying.

Digestive system

Smoking raises the risk of mouth, throat, larynx, and esophagus cancers. People who "smoke but don't inhale" have a higher risk of developing mouth cancer. Smokers are also more likely to develop pancreatic cancer.

Smoking has an influence on insulin, increasing the likelihood of developing insulin resistance. This puts you at a higher risk of developing type 2 diabetes and associated complications, which develop faster in smokers than in nonsmokers.

Reproductive system and sexuality

Nicotine affects both males' and women's sexual blood flow. This can harm men's sexual performance and cause sexual unhappiness in women by reducing lubrication and the capacity to achieve orgasm. Both men and women may have reduced amounts of sex hormones due to smoking. This may result in a decline in sexual desire.

Smoking affects everyone

Smoking impacts not only you but everyone in your life. By quitting smoking, you're doing something good for both yourself and them.

The Effects of Smoking on Your Partner

Most importantly, stopping smoking is a positive step toward better health. As a result, your partner won't have to worry about the long-term health concerns of smoking.

Your lover is sure to appreciate the fact that you no longer have smoker's breath. Another cause of halitosis is gum disease, which is caused by smoking.

It's also true that stopping smoking can help you become more fertile. Nonsmokers, on average, have an easier time conceiving than smokers and are thus more likely to give birth to a healthy baby.

Quitting smoking will save you money, which could be a bonus for your partner. You'll have some more cash to spend on dining out or family vacations.

The Effects of Smoking on Your Children

Children and families are major motivators for smokers to quit. According to a recent poll, 98 percent of children wish their parents would quit smoking, and nearly half of those polled stated their parents' smoking made them sick.

At school, students learn about the consequences of smoking. They are most likely concerned about your health. If you smoke near your children, passive, second-hand smoke may endanger their health.

Smoking puts those closest to you at risk for cancer, heart disease, meningitis, bronchitis, and pneumonia, among other disorders. Second-hand smoke, in fact, raises the risk of lung cancer and heart disease in nonsmokers. The truth is that there is no such thing as a "safe" level of secondhand smoke exposure.

You're helping to establish a smoke-free atmosphere for your friends and family when you quit smoking. This will benefit the health of your family members, particularly children. Furthermore, by making the decision to stop smoking, you will reduce the likelihood of your children taking up the habit.

Consider the extra family outings you'll be able to enjoy with the money you'll save by quitting - days out, trips to the movies, or perhaps that dream family vacation. The benefits of stopping smoking will benefit you all.

How Do You Affect Your Friends If You Smoke?

Don't you despise it when you're having a drink or a meal with pals and then you rush outside to have a cigarette? You're alone outside, missing out on the festivities.

Your friends will be pleased if you go since they care about you and will be able to spend more time with you if you do.

How Smoking Affects Colleagues at Work

It's easy to seek solace by sneaking out of the office for a cigarette break when you're weary, anxious, and up against deadlines. According to studies, smokers can spend up to five weeks away from their workstations, taking 'quick' breaks over the course of a year.

Nobody wants to be accused of not contributing their fair share. Quitting smoking can help you get more done in a day.

Chapter Two

SMOKING: WHAT YOU SHOULD KNOW

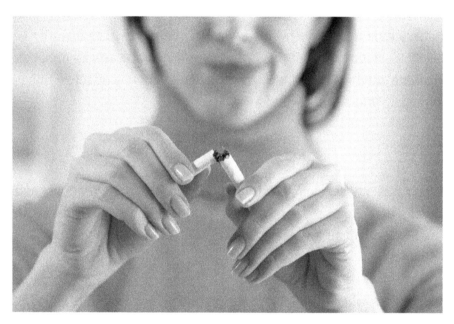

M any ex-smokers claim that quitting Smoking was the most difficult thing they've ever done. Yet, despite this, millions of people have succeeded—and you can, too.

Why Is It So Difficult To Quit?

Learning why you feel the desire to smoke is one of the first stages. You can prepare yourself to find the best techniques to quit smoking after you understand why you smoke. Create a Quit Plan to assist you in identifying your smoking triggers, learn how to manage cravings, and experiment with different quitting techniques.

Withdrawal

Nicotine is one of the key reasons smokers continue to smoke. Nicotine is a substance found in cigarettes that causes addiction. Your body becomes accustomed to nicotine over time. The more you smoke, though, the more nicotine you require to feel normal. As a result, you may feel uneasy and crave cigarettes if your body does not acquire enough nicotine. This is referred to as withdrawal.

It takes time to recover from withdrawal symptoms. The majority of physical symptoms fade after a few days to a week, although cigarette cravings may linger. Nevertheless, you may do a few things to prepare yourself for withdrawal.

Triggers

When you smoke, you associate specific activities, sensations, and people with your smoking. These could "trigger" your desire to smoke. Anticipate smoking triggers and devise strategies to deal with them:

Visit places where Smoking is not permitted. For example, smoking is no longer permitted in many stores, movie theaters, and restaurants.

Spend more time with people who do not smoke. When you're around folks who don't smoke, you won't desire to smoke as much.

Keep your hands occupied at all times. Squeeze a stress ball, play a phone game, or have a healthy snack.

Take a deep breath in and out. Remind yourself of why you want to give up smoking. Then, consider the people in your life who will be happier and healthier as a result of your decision.

How to Recognize Your Smoking Triggers

You're addicted to nicotine, but you're also addicted to the habit of Smoking when you wake up, with a hot drink, after a meal, with alcohol, after sex when you're stressed or weary, hungry or sad, and so on. It's critical to become aware of all the habits you associate with smoking before truly quitting. This practice will help you identify your smoking triggers and break the habits that go along with them. Consider all of the things you do while smoking and imagine doing them while snapping your fingers instead. It felt like something was missing when you tried to execute those tasks without snapping your fingers. We are creatures of habit, so when our routine is disrupted, it can feel uncomfortable at first.

Begin by keeping a week's worth of diaries, noting every time you smoke. Next, make a note on your phone of the many situations in which you smoke, and then place a 1 next to each one every time you smoke in that situation.

Add up how many cigarettes you smoked in each situation after a week. Your list may look something like this:

7: after I wake up

14: after a meal

16: with a hot beverage

5: if you drink alcohol

14: in the car

3: after sex

5: When I'm under pressure

10: Taking a work break

3: when on the Phone

7: before bedtime

5: When I spend time out with_____,

In this case, the most common habit associated with smoking is consuming a hot beverage. My advice is to avoid smoking with a hot beverage for the next few days. After that, for a half-hour, after you eat, don't smoke. After that, quit Smoking in the car or when on the phone.

This will assist you in breaking your links between smoking and specific activities and situations. Try to get to the point where when you do have a cigarette, all you do is smoke it, without the associated habits, in the weeks leading up to your quit date.

Several free quit-smoking applications and websites can assist you in identifying your triggers. These apps also keep track of how many cigarettes you've smoked or not smoked, as well as how much money you save if you quit.

Use a quit-smoking program if you want to quit smoking.

Quit smoking programs assist smokers in understanding and overcoming the challenges they face when attempting to quit.

Problem-solving and other coping skills are taught in the programs. A smoking cessation program can assist you in quitting for good by:

Assisting you in comprehending why you smoke.

You'll learn how to deal with withdrawal and stress.

You'll learn how to fight the impulse to smoke.

Benefits of Quitting Smoking and a Suggested Timeline

Are you ready to give up smoking?

Smoking has several severe health consequences, including an increased chance of major diseases like cancer and heart disease. It can also result in premature death.

While these dangers are a solid reason to quit, withdrawal symptoms can make quitting difficult for some people. Irritability, headaches, and strong nicotine cravings are some of the symptoms.

Although quitting smoking can be difficult, your physical and emotional health rewards are well worth the effort.

What are the advantages?

The cycle of addiction will be broken.

The numerous nicotine receptors in your brain will return to normal within a month of quitting, stopping the cycle of addiction.

Improved circulation

At 2 to 12 weeks of quitting smoking, your blood circulation improves. Physical exercise becomes easier as a result, and your risk of heart attack is reduced.

Improved odor and taste

Smoking damages the nerve endings in your nose and mouth, dulling your senses of taste and smell. However, the nerve endings begin to grow, and your perception of taste and smell improve after 48 hours of quitting.

More vitality

Increased oxygen in your body will provide you with greater energy in addition to enhanced breathing and physical activities.

Your immune system will be boosted

Quitting smoking boosts your immune system by improving circulation, increasing oxygen levels, and lowering inflammation, making it simpler to combat colds and other infections.

Teeth and mouth that are cleaner

Smoking causes your teeth to be yellow, gives you foul breath, and puts you at risk for oral infections. You'll notice and feel a difference in your mouth within a week of quitting.

Enhanced sex life

Smoking might hurt your sexual life. For example, lowering vaginal lubrication and orgasm frequency raises the risk of erectile dysfunction in men and leads to female sexual dysfunction.

Cancer risk is reduced

It may take a few years after you quit Smoking to notice a reduction in your risk of cancers like:

- lung cancer
- esophageal cancer
- cancer of the kidneys
- bladder cancer
- pancreatic cancer

Smoking cessation side effects

For some people, the adverse effects of quitting Smoking might be severe. When people are going through withdrawal, they often feel like they have the flu. This is because smoking impacts all of your body's systems. When you stop smoking, your body must adjust to the lack of nicotine.

It's vital to keep in mind that these adverse effects will only last a short time.

Nausea and headaches

Smoking has an impact on all of your body's systems. As the nicotine exits your body, you may experience headaches, nausea, and other physical symptoms.

Hands and feet tingling

You may experience tingling in your hands and feet as your circulation improves.

Sore throat and coughing

As your lungs clear out the mucus and other material created by Smoking, you may experience a cough and sore throat.

Weight gain as a result of increased appetite

When you stop smoking, you gain more energy, boosting your hunger. In addition, some people eat more due to substituting food for cigarettes to avoid the "hand to mouth" habit of Smoking. Both of these factors contribute to weight gain.

Nicotine cravings become strong.

When you smoke, your body develops a nicotine addiction. It will crave it if you don't give it to it. Cravings are at their peak between two and four weeks.

Anger, irritability, and frustration

You're making a significant shift, and your mind and body will need to adjust to the loss of something on which you've become reliant. Unfortunately, this frequently results in frustration and anger.

Constipation

Nicotine has an effect on the small intestine and colon. When you stop using nicotine, your body may become constipated as it adjusts to not having it.

Anxiety, despair, and insomnia.

The cause for this is unknown, although smokers have a higher risk of sadness and anxiety. To feel better, you may smoke. When you stop smoking, you may experience increased anxiety and depression. Insomnia is another prevalent ailment.

Depression is a very serious condition. It's preferable to seek medical help since they may prescribe talk therapy, medicines, or light treatment. Alternative treatments that can be used in conjunction with doctor-prescribed treatment include:

- omega-3 fatty acids
- acupuncture
- Massage therapy
- meditation
- Supplement with St. John's wort and omega-3 fatty acids.

Concentration problems

It can be tough to concentrate at first due to all of the unwanted effects of quitting Smoking.

Mouth feels dry

Dry mouth is frequently caused by Smoking. However, as you adjust, the stress and anxiety associated with withdrawal can make things worse.

Seven other Reasons to Give Up Smoking

- Psoriasis
- Gangrene
- Impotence
- Stroke
- Blindness

- Degenerative disk disease (DDD)
- Other types of cancer

There's more to lung cancer than that.

You're probably aware that smoking cigarettes promote lung cancer and heart problems. You're well aware that it discolors your teeth. It wrinkles your skin, stains your fingers, and dulls your senses of smell and taste, as you're well aware.

However, you have yet to succeed in quitting. So, just in case you're still not convinced, here are seven more not-so-fun side effects of smoking that you may not be aware of.

Psoriasis

This itchy, plaque-skin autoimmune condition is not caused by Smoking. However, researchers are convinced of two things regarding psoriasis: first, it has a hereditary component. Second, according to the National Psoriasis Foundation, smoking cigarettes more than doubles the risk of acquiring psoriasis in people who have the gene.

Gangrene

You've probably heard of gangrene. It happens when tissue in your body decomposes, resulting in foul odors. Gangrene develops when a part of the body receives insufficient blood supply. Smoking for a long time constricts blood vessels and reduces blood flow.

Impotence

Regular, long-term Smoking causes gangrene by constricting blood vessels, and it can also cut off blood supply to male genitalia. Do you think Viagra or Cialis will work for you? Unfortunately, that is not the case. Most erectile dysfunction (E.D.) medications are rendered worthless by the chemical changes that occur in the body due to Smoking.

Stroke

While your blood vessels react to carcinogens, they may also send a potentially fatal blood clot to your brain. Even if the blood clot isn't fatal, it can cause catastrophic brain damage.

Blindness

If you continue to smoke cigarettes, macular degeneration may develop, rendering you blind since smoking obstructs your retina's blood flow. It's also possible that you'll go blind for the rest of your life.

Degenerative disk disease (DDD)

Smoking hastens the degradation of our spines, which were never supposed to live forever. Chronic back pain, herniated disks, and possibly osteoarthritis result from the discs between your vertebrae losing fluid and being unable to effectively protect and support the vertebrae (O.A.).

Other types of cancer

You've probably heard of lung cancer; it's usually the first thing people bring up when they're giving you reasons to quit Smoking. But don't forget about the following cancers:

- the liver, the kidneys, or the bladder

- mouth or lip

- esophagus, laryngeal, or throat

- colon or stomach

- pancreatic

- cervical

Leukemia is also a possibility. The more you smoke, the higher your risk of developing any of these cancers.

Takeaway

If you're ready to give up smoking, there are a variety of options for getting started. It's not an easy task, but with the right advice and aid, it'll get easier by the day.

It's your life, after all. It's all about your health. Make an informed decision.

Chapter Three

SET YOUR SCHEDULE

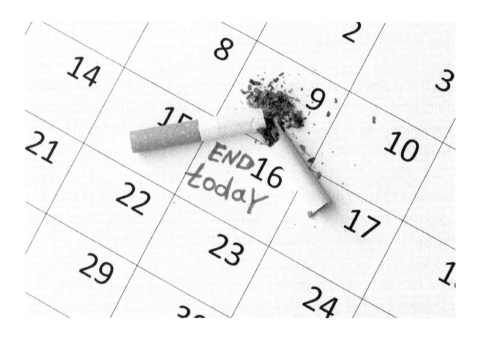

Timeline for quitting Smoking

Your heart rate reduces 20 minutes after you stop smoking. Cigarettes cause your blood pressure to rise and your heart rate to speed up. Within 20 minutes of your last smoke, your heart rate will begin to return to normal.

Your blood carbon monoxide level declines 8 to 12 hours after you quit smoking. Carbon monoxide is the same hazardous gas emitted by automobile exhaust. It increases your heart rate and makes you breathless. The carbon monoxide level in your blood declines, and your blood oxygen level rises within 8 to 12 hours.

Your sense of smell and taste increases 48 hours after you quit smoking. The nerve endings in your nose and mouth that have been destroyed by smoking start to heal, enhancing your sense of smell and taste.

Your risk of heart attack decreases 2 to 3 months after you quit Smoking. Improved circulation, decreased blood pressure, and heart rate, as well as improved oxygen levels and lung function, all lessen your risk of a heart attack.

You'll feel less short of breath and cough in less than 1 to 9 months after quitting. After that, coughing, shortness of breath, and nasal congestion will become less of an issue. Overall, you'll feel more energized.

Your risk of heart disease will be decreased in half after a year of not smoking. But, on the other hand, smoking greatly raises your chances of developing heart disease.

Your risk of stroke lowers after 5 years of not smoking. Within 5 to 15 years of stopping smoking, your risk of stroke will be the same as someone who has never smoked, depending on how much and how long you smoked and your overall health.

Your risk of lung cancer is lowered than that of someone who has never smoked ten years after quitting. Your rate of dying from lung cancer will be the same as someone who has never smoked. Your chances of getting other cancers are greatly reduced.

After quitting smoking for 15 years, your risk of heart disease is the same as someone who has never smoked. In addition, you'll have lower cholesterol, thinner blood (which lowers your chance of blood clots), and lower blood pressure once you quit Smoking.

Smoking cessation vs. vaping cessation

When it comes to smoking, vaping may appear to be the lesser of two evils. Although vaping is less dangerous than smoking, it still contains nicotine and other toxins, many of which are also contained in regular cigarettes.

Even some nicotine-free vapes have been discovered to contain nicotine. For some people, stopping vaping might be just as tough as quitting Smoking.

While some data suggests that vaping may aid in smoking cessation in some persons, the US E-cigarettes have not been approved by the FDA as a smoking cessation tool.

Find a doctor who can assist you with quitting.

A physician can assist you in quitting Smoking. If you're ready to quit, talk to your doctor or find a doctor who can assist you. A doctor can provide you with information on drugs that can assist you in quitting or connect you with local options.

Make a list of all the reasons why you'd like to quit smoking.

Keep the list somewhere you'll see it frequently, like your car or the spot where you used to keep your cigarettes. Take a glance at the list whenever you feel the need to smoke to remind yourself why you want to quit.

The most important reason for you to desire to quit.

Okay, here's the most important reason to give up Smoking: Are you paying attention? Because this is, without a doubt, the most significant thing, I'll say in the entire book. You want to stop Smoking because you value your well-being. You adore yourself, I'll say it again. When you love yourself, you look after and care for yourself. You only feed your body healthy stuff.

Your Life

The most obvious advantage of quitting Smoking is that you will live longer and healthier. Smoking is a leading cause of heart disease and cancer, and it's a life-threatening habit for many people. One-fifth of people in the United States die as a result of smoking-related causes. [ii] Quitting Smoking is the single most effective strategy to live longer (which is why your family wants you to quit).

Your Well-being

Tobacco use can result in life-threatening illnesses. However, many people are unaware of all of the potential health risks associated with Smoking. For example, smoking causes asthma, bad skin, infertility, high blood pressure, sexual disorders (including erectile dysfunction), discolored teeth and gums, and it takes longer to recover from a cold.

Your Sexual life

Smoking increases the risk of erectile dysfunction (E.D.) by about 50% in men in their 30s, 40s, and older, and if you smoke 20 or more cigarettes per day, your risk is 60% higher than if you never smoked. Erections are difficult to achieve unless blood can flow freely into the penis, so these blood vessels must be in good health. It has been established that smoking damages and deteriorates blood vessels. Nicotine narrows the arteries that provide blood to the penis, lowering blood flow and pressure.

This constriction of the blood arteries worsens with time, so if you don't have any symptoms today, they may worsen later. Men who smoke may experience erection problems as an early warning indication that cigarettes are causing damage to other parts of the body, such as the blood arteries that supply the heart. Because Smoking has such a negative impact on a man's sexual performance, the first question doctors ask any man with erectile dysfunction is, "Are you a smoker?"

Your Financial Situation

One of the most wonderful aspects of quitting is that you suddenly find yourself with more money. You may use the money you spend on cigarettes towards other things, giving you a lot more spare cash. In any event, you're squandering hundreds of dollars per month that could be put to far better use.

Your schedule

You won't need to arrange smoke breaks once you quit Smoking. The average smoker smokes for 1 hour every day. So you won't have to be concerned with cigarette scheduling or when you'll be able to squeeze them in once you've quit. Instead, consider how you could put that extra hour in your day to good use.

Your Substance Abuse

Tobacco is one of the most addicting substances we've ever encountered. Getting rid of that monkey off your back requires quitting. It entails a complete absence of cravings and withdrawal symptoms. It is empowering to have control over your life and conduct.

Embarrassment in Public

Nowadays, smokers have a poor reputation. Smoking used to be associated with sophistication, but now it is associated with filthy, stinky people who are addicted to a repulsive habit. Smokers face explicit discrimination, with some employers refusing to hire them if they smoke. When you stop, you are no longer stigmatized. Non-smokers find the odor disgusting.

People may not say anything, but smokers have a unique stench, similar to terrible body odor, repulsive to non-smokers. Second-hand Smoke Studies have revealed that second-hand smoke is far more hazardous than previously believed. If you smoke at home, you are endangering your family's health. Secondhand smoke is unfiltered, making it possibly more harmful, even if it is not inhaled directly. Smoke can remain in a room for hours after you've put out the cigarette, even if you're not smoking in front of people.

Your Children and Family

According to studies, children of smokers are significantly more likely to become smokers themselves. There isn't a single smoker in the world who would wish the habit on their children, no matter how much they enjoy smoking. According to studies, children of smokers are more likely to have behavioral issues and have challenges in school.

Maintaining a smoke-free household and informing your children about the harms of Smoking will assist, but quitting Smoking can help much more—finally, the most compelling reason of all. Your family will be delighted to see you succeed. When you quit, you feel as if you've been given a new lease on life and a great sense of accomplishment.

Chapter Four

UNDERSTAND NICOTINE WITHDRAWAL

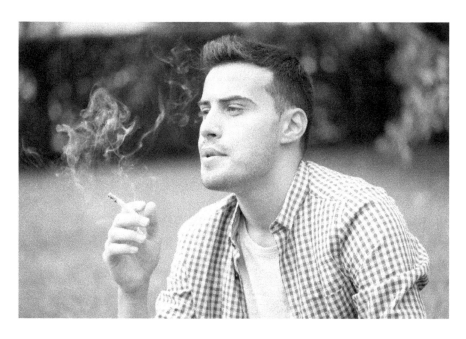

What is nicotine withdrawal, and how does it happen?

S moking is addicting because of the chemical nicotine, which is frequently connected with tobacco. It can affect the brain in a variety of ways, including:

- uplifting the mood

- depression alleviation
- irritability reduction
- improving short-term memory and attention
- generating a feeling of well-being
- appetite suppression

Like alcohol, cocaine, and morphine, Nicotine can be extremely addictive.

Tobacco is known to contain around 70 carcinogens in addition to nicotine. Smoking-related disorders such as lung cancer, heart disease, and stroke can all be caused by these substances.

Every year, millions of smokers try to quit to avoid these ailments. As of 2015, 68 percent of smokers said they wanted to quit fully, according to the Centers for Disease Control and Prevention.

Nicotine withdrawal makes quitting even more difficult.

What are the signs and symptoms of nicotine withdrawal?

Nicotine withdrawal symptoms might appear as soon as 30 minutes after you last used tobacco, depending on your level of addiction. The severity of your symptoms will be influenced by how long you smoked cigarettes and how much tobacco you consume daily.

For smokers, nicotine withdrawal symptoms include:

- a strong desire for nicotine
- tingle in the palms and soles of the feet
- sweating
- nausea and stomach cramps

- gas and constipation
- headaches
- coughing
- throat irritation
- insomnia
- concentration problems
- anxiety
- irritability
- depression
- gaining weight

Chewing tobacco users experience withdrawal symptoms that are quite similar to those of smokers. They are as follows:

- a depressed state of mind
- sleeping problems
- concentration problems
- feeling jittery and restless
- irritability
- hunger pangs or weight gain
- a reduced heart rate

Nicotine withdrawal symptoms usually peak in two to three days.

Nicotine receptors in the brain are the source of your cravings. These receptors have become more active as a result of your earlier nicotine use. You'll want to keep Smoking because of the receptors. Withdrawal symptoms occur when certain receptors are ignored.

However, as you ignore them, they gradually fade away. Withdrawal symptoms usually subside after two to four weeks. Nicotine withdrawal can last several months in some people.

What is the treatment for nicotine withdrawal?

If you decide to stop smoking, talk to your doctor about dealing with the withdrawal symptoms. They might be able to help you get access to prescription medication or information about local support groups.

Nicotine withdrawal can be treated using a variety of approaches. They are as follows:

Nicotine replacement therapy (NRT) is available over-the-counter (OTC). Nicotine gum and skin patches are two examples.

Nicotine replacement therapy on prescription. Inhalers and nasal sprays are two examples.

These can help alleviate symptoms by gradually lowering nicotine levels in the body.

Non-nicotine prescription drugs, such as bupropion (Zyban) or varenicline, may be used as part of the treatment.

Nicotine replacement therapy (NRT) is beneficial, but it is not a cure. The majority of people still have withdrawal symptoms. In addition, NRT will not be able to remove your emotional attachment to Smoking.

NRT's benefits and drawbacks

The following are some of the most prevalent side effects of popular NRT products:

- dizziness

- sleeping problems

- nausea

- headaches

However, most researchers have found that the risks of using NRT outweigh the benefits. As a result, many insurance plans cover it.

Although NRT products have been linked to higher blood pressure, a 2016 study found that NRT is unlikely to raise blood pressure.

Although some people have had heart attacks while using a nicotine patch and smoking simultaneously, blood pressure increases due to the increased nicotine from both sources, not the patch. As a result, it is unlikely to raise blood pressure when the patch is properly applied.

If your blood pressure rises, check with your doctor to ensure you're on the proper medication.

Quitting cold turkey.

People who smoke more than ten cigarettes per day should use NRT. If you only smoke ten cigarettes a day or less, you may want to try stopping "cold turkey," which is quitting without using nicotine replacements. Your withdrawal symptoms will be more severe, but having a plan in place will help you get through it. The following suggestions may assist you in successfully quitting:

- Set a date for quitting smoking. This is best done when you don't have a lot on your schedule.

- Make a list of the reasons you want to stop.

- Remind yourself that the symptoms of withdrawal are just temporary.

- Seek the help of friends and relatives.

- Become a member of a support group.

If you're attempting to quit smoking, you might find it helpful to ask for aid from those who are also trying to quit. Participating in a smoking cessation program or a support group can help you succeed.

What are some of the side effects of quitting smoking?

Nicotine withdrawal does not pose a risk of death. However, once you stop smoking, you may experience certain physical or mental changes.

Weight gain and increased hunger

Your taste buds and sense of smell will return to normal once you stop smoking. While this is a good thing, you may find that you crave food more frequently than you did before starting smoking. Additionally, some people start to seek high-fat, high-sugar foods, even if they didn't before they started smoking.

The following suggestions will help you manage your cravings and lose weight:

Food craving

- Delay your cravings for a few minutes, drink a glass of water, distract yourself with anything else, or practice deep breathing by practicing the "four Ds."

- Snack on carrots, raw almonds, or low-fat yogurt for a nutritious snack.

- Use a toothpick or a straw to keep your hands and mouth occupied.

- Slow down your eating. Take pleasure in the flavors of your cuisine.

- Avoid watching T.V. or other forms of distraction while eating. Instead, recognize when you're hungry and when you're simply bored.

- Exercise. Even a little walk around the block can assist you in losing weight.

- If you're worried about your weight, talk to your health care physician. They may be able to help you.

Changes in mental health

Mental health difficulties may also be present in some people. For example, people who have previously experienced depression may experience a recurrence. People who have experienced bipolar disorder or other substance use disorders may also experience this.

Nicotine withdrawal depression is usually very temporary and passes with time. Depression is a treatable disorder, but it can be life-threatening if left untreated. If you suffer from depression, ask your doctor about coping with your symptoms while stopping.

How to deal with nicotine withdrawal

You'll suffer nicotine withdrawal whether you quit cold turkey or with NRT. But, even though you won't be able to avoid it, you will be able to navigate your way through it. Some ways of dealing with the most prevalent withdrawal symptoms are listed below.

Sore throat and dry mouth

- Drink plenty of water, chew sugarless gum, or eat sugarless candy

Headaches

• Take a bath or do deep breathing exercises. You can also use over-the-counter pain relievers like ibuprofen (Advil) or acetaminophen (Tylenol).

Sleeping problems

• One to two hours before night, turn off or put away electronic gadgets. Make a bedtime ritual out of reading, showering or having a nice bath, or listening to relaxing music. Before bed, drink a glass of herbal tea or warm milk and avoid caffeine and heavy meals.

Concentration problems

• Take a lot of breaks. Make sure you don't overdo it. Make to-do lists and provide plenty of time for chores to be completed.

What are the long-term prospects?

The most difficult element of stopping Smoking is usually overcoming nicotine withdrawal. Many people have to try to quit multiple times. The more you try to quit, the better your chances are of succeeding.

After the withdrawal symptoms have passed, you may still have long-term cravings for tobacco. For long-term success, you'll need to control your cravings.

• Many people can control their cravings by avoiding triggers, exercising moderately, and doing deep breathing exercises. In addition, cravings can be reduced by finding ways to relax, such as:Play some music.

Take up a new hobby.

• Take a stroll.

- Consult your friends and relatives.

- Another useful idea is to replace smokes with carrots, gum, or hard candy. These can help to reduce the psychological desire to smoke.

Chapter Five

HYPNOSIS TO QUIT SMOKING

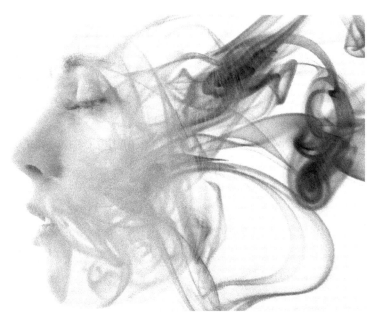

U nderstandably, so many people desire to stop smoking. Yet, according to a 2019 research review, it is the world's leading cause of preventable illness and death.

Stopping smoking can improve your health, but quitting is difficult for many people. There are a variety of strategies and products available to help you quit smoking. Hypnosis receives a lot of attention.

Some people attribute their success to hypnosis. However, studies have produced contradictory results, indicating that more research is required.

When used in conjunction with other smoking cessation methods, hypnotherapy is likely to assist some people in quitting smoking.

If you want to attempt this or any other strategy, talk to your doctor about it. They can help you come up with a plan that works for you.

What exactly is hypnosis?

Hypnosis has long been utilized for entertainment purposes. It appears to be a form of mind control in that circumstance. The hypnotist exerts control over the subject and encourages them to engage in irrational behavior. But it's only for show.

Hypnotherapy is real, but it does not include mind control. It's more of a contemplative state at this point.

A professional hypnotist employs verbal cues to guide you into a concentrated, meditative state in which you may be more receptive to suggestions. The therapist will make recommendations depending on your objectives.

Unlike the audience members in those theatrical productions, you will not be hypnotized. You can't be forced to do anything you don't want to do.

Hypnosis has the potential to help people quit smoking.

It's possible that hypnosis alone won't be enough to help you stop smoking for good. However, it might be useful to:

- Make smoking less appealing to you.
- bolster your desire to stop
- assist you in staying focused on your smoking cessation plan

Hypnosis can help you quit by reinforcing what you're already doing.

When paired with other treatments, hypnosis can improve the effectiveness of other treatments, according to a 2017 study review reviewing developments in hypnosis research.

According to the review, limited evidence suggests that hypnotherapy may be effective for various conditions, including smoking.

A 2008 randomized trial found that hypnosis combined with nicotine patches compares favorably to standard behavioral counseling for long-term quitting.

However, according to a 2019 research review, when it comes to hypnosis and smoking cessation:

- Hypnotists might exaggerate their success rates.
- Positive findings in uncontrolled studies may not be indicative of long-term success.

There isn't enough research to indicate whether hypnotherapy is more successful than other counseling methods or self-suicide.

Is there any danger in using hypnosis to quit smoking?

There is no proof that hypnotherapy has any negative consequences or is hazardous in any manner. If you place all your hopes in it, though, you may be disappointed.

If you want to quit Smoking and are interested in hypnotherapy, you should consider incorporating it into a larger plan. First, consult a doctor for assistance in stopping Smoking.

What does smoking cessation hypnotherapy look like?

Smoking cessation is complex, and a few hypnotic suggestions won't help. Know what you need to succeed in hypnotherapy:

- a willingness to learn attitude
- patience
- determination

At your first appointment, you'll discuss your smoking habits and your desire to quit. What you've tried so far and what methods you'll continue to work on alongside hypnosis should also be discussed.

Methods of hypnotherapy may differ slightly from one therapist to the next, so ask potential therapists how they plan to go about it.

Sessions might last anywhere between 60 and 90 minutes. The number of sessions required is determined by how well you respond to hypnosis and how much reinforcement you believe you require.

Using verbal cues and mental pictures, your hypnotherapist will take you to a peaceful, meditative state. You'll get suggestions like these while you're in this altered level of awareness:

- Smoking is harmful to your health.
- When you smoke, you don't feel well.
- Smoke should be avoided at all costs.
- You should exercise control over your smoking rather than allowing smoking to control you.

- As a non-smoker, you'll have a lot of advantages.

When the impulse to smoke strikes, it serves as a reminder of healthier alternatives.

The idea is for these thoughts to come to mind whenever you feel the need to smoke. Remember, you'll be completely aware of everything that's going on. You will not lose control of your actions during or after the session.

The therapist may also do the following to help you remember what you've learned:

- give audio or video recordings that can be listened to or watched at home
- Apps that you can utilize on your own
- instruct you on the fundamentals of self-hypnosis

According to a 2019 review, self-hypnosis for quitting smoking is linked to a 20 to 35 percent 6-month abstinence rate.

How much does hypnotherapy for smoking cessation cost?

Individual practitioners and locales have different prices.

The American Association of Professional Hypnotherapists estimates that smoking cessation sessions cost $75 to $125 each session. Some of them may be even higher.

All health insurance policies do not cover hypnotherapy. When you hire a skilled specialist, several insurance companies may cover a portion of the cost.

To avoid being taken off guard, verify your policy or call your insurance carrier before booking an appointment.

If you're worried about the price, it's a good idea to talk about it right away. Inquire about self-hypnosis and other tools that you can use at home.

What is the best place to look for a professional?

If you're looking for hypnosis to help you quit smoking, here are a few places to start your search:

- Consult your physician.
- Enlist the help of people you know for referrals.
- Consult your health insurance provider.

Local mental health and human service agencies should be contacted.

Hypnotherapists and mental health professionals should contact professional associations.

Before making an appointment, schedule an arrangement to chat with the hypnotherapist.

Because hypnosis requires you to relax and enter a meditative state, it's critical that you feel at ease with the hypnotherapist and find their voice comforting.

Things to talk about ahead of time:

- Qualifications and training
- experience in assisting smokers in quitting

- whether or not they will offer you materials to use on your own

You may be asked to commit to a certain number of sessions by some hypnotists. You should generally hold off on purchasing a whole package until you've had a chance to try out a session.

Do hypnosis applications for quitting smoking work?

There isn't a lot of scientific evidence that hypnosis apps can help you quit smoking. Because hypnosis is challenging to study, much of what we hear is based on anecdotal evidence.

On the other hand, there is an increasing number of quit-smoking applications on the market, and a significant number of them use self-hypnosis as a strategy. You can use these apps on their own or in conjunction with hypnotherapy.

In a 2020 clinical trial, two approaches to quit-smoking apps were compared. One is based on U.S. clinical practice guidelines (USCPG), which involves avoiding things that make you want to smoke.

Acceptance and commitment therapy is another approach to quit-smoking apps. This is a mindful approach in which you recognize triggers and alter your response.

In the ACT app group, the chances of quitting Smoking were 1.49 times higher.

Alternative Treatments for quitting Smoking

There are many different ways to quit smoking, and there is no one-size-fits-all solution. It may take a few tries to figure out what works best for you. The following are a few examples of these techniques:

- Cognitive-behavioral therapy (CBT)

- Nicotine patches, gum, and lozenges

- varenicline, a non-nicotine prescription medication

- Acupuncture and meditation are examples of complementary therapies.

- cold turkey or gradual withdrawal

Hypnosis is a therapeutic tool that can help people with various issues, including quitting Smoking.

If you want to try hypnosis to quit smoking, make sure you find a qualified practitioner with smoking cessation experience.

You must be open to hypnosis and comfortable with your hypnotherapist for it to work.

Although there isn't much evidence to support its effectiveness, there's little risk in using it as part of a comprehensive smoking cessation strategy.

Fact vs. fiction: 6 popular myths debunked

Many myths about hypnosis persist, even though it slowly becomes more accepted in traditional medical practices. Here, we distinguish between truth and lies.

Myth: Hypnosis is a practice everyone can undergo.

Not everyone can be hypnotized. According to one study, about 10% of the population is highly hypnotizable. Although the rest of the population could be hypnotized, they are less likely to accept the technique.

Myth: When people are hypnotized, they lose control of their bodies.

During hypnosis, you have complete control over your body. You'll remain aware of what you're doing and what's being asked of you despite what you see with stage hypnosis. You won't do something you don't want to do under hypnosis if you don't want to.

Myth: Hypnosis and sleep are the same things.

You may appear to be sleeping during hypnosis, but you are actually awake. You're just in a deep state of relaxation. You may become drowsy as your muscles become limp and your breathing rate slows.

Myth: When people are hypnotized, they can't lie.

Hypnotism isn't a cure-all for truth. You have more openness to suggestions during hypnosis, but you still have free will and moral judgment. You can't be forced to say anything you don't want to say, whether it's a lie or not.

Myth: You can be hypnotized while surfing the web.

Many smartphone apps and Internet videos promote Self-hypnosis, but they are likely ineffective.

These tools aren't usually created by a certified hypnotist or hypnosis organization, according to researchers in a 2013 review. Doctors and hypnotists advise against using them because of this.

Hypnosis can help you "recover" lost memories, but this is probably a myth.

While it is possible to retrieve memories while in hypnosis, you are also more likely to create false memories while in this state. As a result, many hypnotists are hesitant to use hypnosis for memory retrieval.

In conclusion

Hypnosis has all the stereotypes of a stage show, with clucking chickens and daring dancers.

On the other hand, hypnosis is a legitimate therapeutic therapy that can be used to cure various ailments. Insomnia, depression, and pain management are all examples of this.

It's critical to work with a professional hypnotist or hypnotherapist if you want to be confident in the guided hypnosis process. They will devise a strategy to assist you in achieving your specific objectives.

Chapter Six

HOW TO FIGHT TOBACCO CRAVINGS

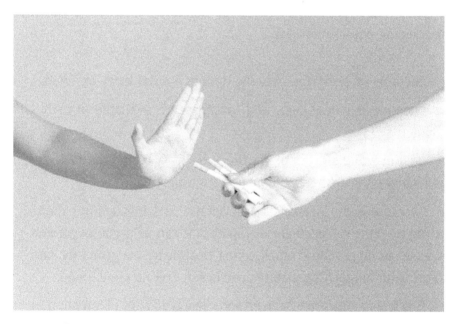

When you're attempting to quit Smoking, cravings for tobacco might be exhausting. To reduce and resist cravings, follow these guidelines.

Tobacco cravings or urges to smoke can be strong for most tobacco users. Your desires, on the other hand, have no power over you.

When you have a strong desire to use tobacco, remember that, no matter how strong the desire is, it will pass in five to ten minutes whether you smoke a cigarette or chew a piece of chewing tobacco. So you're one step closer to quitting tobacco use for good each time you overcome a cigarette need.

Here are ten techniques to help you resist the urge to smoke or use tobacco when you have a tobacco need.

Use a nicotine replacement product.

Inquire with your physician about nicotine replacement therapy. Among the possibilities are:

- Nicotine on prescription in the form of a nasal spray or inhaler
- Nicotine patches, gum, and lozenges are available over-the-counter.
- Non-nicotine stop-smoking drugs such as bupropion (Zyban) and varenicline are available on prescription (Chantix)
- Nicotine gum, lozenges, nasal sprays, and inhalers are short-acting nicotine replacement therapies that can help you overcome intense cravings. These quick-acting treatments are generally safe to use with long-acting nicotine patches or non-nicotine drugs.
- Electronic cigarettes have recently received a lot of attention as a viable replacement for regular cigarettes. However, more research is needed to determine the efficacy of electronic cigarettes for smoking cessation and their long-term safety.

Stay away from potential triggers

When you're in situations where you frequently smoke or chew tobacco, such as at parties or bars, or when you're anxious or sipping coffee, your tobacco cravings are likely to be the strongest.

Determine your trigger situations and design a plan to avoid or overcome them without the use of tobacco.

Don't put yourself in a scenario where you'll have to reintroduce smoking. If you used to smoke while talking on the phone, for example, keep a pen and paper nearby so you may doodle instead of Smoking.

Get some exercise

Physical activity can assist in diverting your attention away from tobacco cravings and lower the strength of those cravings. Even small bursts of physical exercise, such as sprinting up and down the stairs a few times, can help you get rid of your tobacco urge. Take a walk or jog outside.

Try squats, deep knee bends, pushups, sprinting in place, or walking up and down a flight of stairs if you're stuck at home or work. If exercise isn't your thing, try prayer, embroidery, woodworking, or journaling. Alternatively, undertake household duties like sweeping or filing documents to keep yourself occupied.

Postponement

If you're about to succumb to your cigarette need, remind yourself that you must first wait 10 minutes — and then do anything to occupy your time at that time. Try going to a smoke-free public area. These basic techniques may be sufficient to quell your cigarette need.

Work on your relaxation skills

Smoking could have been a coping mechanism for you when you were stressed. Resisting a cigarette addiction can be hard in and of itself. Relaxation practices, such as deep breathing exercises, muscular relaxation, yoga, visualization, massage, or listening to relaxing music, can help relieve stress.

Chew it up

To combat a cigarette craving, give your tongue something to do. Chew sugarless gum or hard candies, or eat raw carrots, celery, almonds, or sunflower seeds for a pleasing crunch.

Don't have 'just one.'

To satisfy a tobacco appetite, you could be tempted to smoke just one cigarette. But don't kid yourself into thinking you'll be able to stop there. Having just one usually leads to another, and you may find yourself smoking again.

Look for help on the internet.

Participate in an online quit-smoking program. Alternatively, read a quitter's blog and leave supportive comments for someone who is battling cigarette cravings. Learn from other people's experiences with tobacco addiction.

Request reinforcements

Make contact with a family member, a friend, or a support group member for assistance in resisting a tobacco addiction. Call each other, go for a stroll together, have a few laughs, or get together to commiserate about your hunger pangs.

Remind yourself of the advantages.

To overcome cigarette cravings, write down or express out loud the reasons you want to quit smoking. For example, these could include the following:

- I'm feeling much better now.

- Getting in better shape

- Keeping your loved ones from being exposed to secondhand smoke

- saving money

Remember that doing something to overcome an impulse is always preferable to doing nothing. And every time you resist a cigarette need, you're one step closer to quitting smoking for good.

Chapter Seven

HOW TO QUIT SMOKING

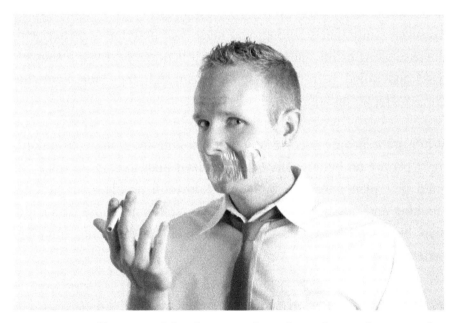

W e're all aware of the dangers of smoking, but it doesn't make quitting any easier. Whether you're a once-in-a-while teen smoker or a lifelong pack-a-day smoker, quitting is difficult.

Tobacco use is both a physical and psychological addiction. Cigarettes contain nicotine, which delivers a short-term — and addictive — high. When you stop getting your nicotine fix, your body goes through physical withdrawal symptoms and craves. You may resort to cigarettes as a quick and reliable way to improve your mood, relieve stress, and unwind due to nicotine's "feel good" influence on the brain. However, smoking can also cope with despair, anxiety, and boredom. Finding new, healthier methods to cope with those sensations is part of quitting.

It is also established that smoking is a daily practice. Smoking a cigarette with your morning coffee, at a break at work or school, or on your trip home at the end of a long day may be an automatic response for you. Perhaps your friends, relatives, or coworkers smoke, and it's been ingrained in your interactions with them.

To successfully quit smoking, you must treat both the addiction and the associated habits and routines. But it is possible. Even if they've tried and failed before, any smoker can kick the habit with the correct support and quit strategy.

While some people successfully quit smoking by going cold turkey, most people do better with a personalized plan to stay on track. A solid quit plan considers both the short-term problem of quitting smoking and the long-term challenge of avoiding relapse. It should also be adapted to your individual requirements and smoking patterns.

Self-examination questions

Consider what kind of smoker you are, as well as when and why you require a cigarette. This will assist you in determining which advice, approaches, or therapies are most appropriate for you.

Are you a daily smoker who consumes more than a pack of cigarettes? Or do you like to smoke in public? Is it possible to quit with just a nicotine patch?

Do you have any activities, places, or persons in mind that you associate with Smoking? For example, do you feel compelled to smoke after each meal or anytime you have a coffee break?

When you're anxious or depressed, do you go for a cigarette? Is your cigarette smoking linked to other vices like drinking or gambling?

Discover the START method

S = Set a deadline for quitting.

Choose a date within the next two weeks so you can prepare without losing motivation to quit. For example, if you smoke mostly at work, try quitting over the weekend, so you have a few days to acclimate.

T = Inform your family, friends, and coworkers that you intend to quit.

Tell your friends and family about your plan to quit smoking and that you'll need their help and encouragement. Look for a quit buddy who is also trying to quit smoking. You can assist one other in getting through difficult times.

A = Anticipate and prepare for the obstacles you'll encounter while quitting.

Most of those who re-start Smoking do it within the first three months. However, you can make it easier on yourself by anticipating frequent problems like nicotine withdrawal and cigarette cravings.

R = Get rid of cigarettes and other tobacco products from your home, car, and place of business.

T = Speak with your doctor about quitting aid.

To aid with withdrawal symptoms, your doctor may prescribe medicine. If you can't see a doctor, several over-the-counter medications, such as nicotine patches, lozenges, and gum, are available at your local drugstore.

Find out what makes you want to smoke.

Identifying the things that make you want to smoke, such as specific events, activities, feelings, and people, is one of the finest things you can do to help yourself quit.

Keep a journal of your cravings.

A craving journal can aid in the identification of trends and triggers. Keep a smoking log for the week or so leading up to your quit date. Keep track of the times during the day that you crave a cigarette:

- What time was it, exactly?
- On a scale of one to ten, how strong was the desire?
- So, what were you up to?
- Who were you with at the time?
- What were your thoughts at the time?
- After you smoked, how did you feel?
- Do you smoke to get rid of bad feelings?

Many people smoke to cope with negative emotions like stress, depression, loneliness, and worry. When you're having a rough day, cigarettes may seem like your only friend. However, as relaxing as cigarettes are, it's vital to realize healthier and more effective ways to manage negative emotions. Exercising, meditating, relaxation techniques, and basic breathing exercises are examples of these.

Finding other strategies to deal with tough feelings without turning to cigarettes is vital to quitting smoking. However, even if cigarettes are no longer a part of your life, the painful and unpleasant sensations that drove you to smoke in the first place will linger. So it's worth devoting some time to pondering how you plan to handle difficult situations and minor irritations that would normally set you off.

Tips on how to avoid common triggers

Alcohol. When individuals drink, many of them smoke. Switch to non-alcoholic beverages or drink solely in venues where Smoking is not permitted inside. Snacking on nuts, sucking on a straw, or chewing on a cocktail stick are some options.

Others who smoke. It's even more difficult to quit or avoid relapse when your friends, family, and coworkers smoke. Tell people about your decision to quit smoking, so they know they won't be able to smoke with you in the car or during a coffee break. Find non-smokers to chat with during your breaks at work or do something else, like go for a stroll.

End of a meal. For some smokers, finishing a meal involves lighting up, and the notion of quitting Smoking might be intimidating. You can, however, substitute something different for that time after a meal, such as a piece of fruit, a nutritious dessert, a square of chocolate, or a stick of gum.

Managing the effects of nicotine withdrawal

When you stop smoking, your body will likely experience various physical symptoms as it adjusts to the lack of nicotine in your system. Nicotine withdrawal sets up immediately within an hour of the last cigarette and lasts two to three days. Depending on the individual, withdrawal symptoms can last anywhere from a few days to several weeks.

Some of the most prevalent nicotine withdrawal symptoms are listed here:

- Cravings for cigarettes
- Irritability, frustration, or anger
- Nervousness or anxiety
- Concentration problems
- Restlessness
- Appetite increase
- Headaches
- Insomnia
- Tremors
- increased Coughing.
- Fatigue
- Constipation or a stomach ache
- Depression
- lowered Heart rate.

It's crucial to remember that these withdrawal symptoms are just temporary, as terrible as they are. They will improve in a few weeks when the toxins are cleared from your body. Meanwhile, inform your friends and family that you might not be your usual self and beg for their patience.

Control your cigarette cravings

While avoiding smoking triggers will help minimize your desire to smoke, you are unlikely to be able to completely avoid cigarette cravings. Cravings, fortunately, don't last long—usually 5 to 10 minutes. If you're tempted to smoke, tell yourself that the urge will pass quickly and strive to resist. It is good to plan ahead of time and have techniques in place to deal with cravings.

Distract yourself from the situation. Dishwashing, watching T.V., showering, or calling a buddy are all options. It doesn't matter what you do as long as you're not thinking about Smoking.

Remind yourself why you chose to quit. Concentrate on your reasons for quitting, like health benefits (for example, lowering your risk of heart disease and lung cancer), improved appearances, money saved, and increased self-esteem.

Get yourself out of a tempting position. The need could be triggered by where you are or what you're doing. If that's the case, a change of environment can make a world of difference.

Reward yourself for your efforts. Make a point of reinforcing your accomplishments. For example, give yourself a gift whenever you defeat a craving to keep yourself motivated.

Dealing with immediate cigarette cravings

Find an oral alternative - Have other items on hand to pop into your mouth when you get a craving. Mints, sunflower seeds, celery sticks, gum, or carrot are all good options. Alternatively, suck on a drinking straw.

Listen to music you like while reading a book or magazine, solve a crossword or Sudoku puzzle, or play an online game to keep your mind occupied.

Occupy your hands – Squeeze balls, pencils, and paper clips are all wonderful options for satisfying the tactile stimulation need.

Brush your teeth — The fresh, clean feeling can help you resist smoking.

Drink water - Drink a large glass of water slowly. Staying hydrated will not only help you get rid of the need, but it will also help you avoid the unpleasant side effects of nicotine withdrawal.

Light anything else instead of a cigarette - a candle or some incense will suffice.

Stroll, do some jumping jacks or pushups, attempt some yoga stretches, or run around the block to get some exercise.

Relax by doing something calming, such as taking a warm bath, meditating, reading a book, or practicing deep breathing techniques.

Enter a public building, store, mall, coffee shop, or movie theater, for example, where smoking is prohibited.

How to avoid gaining weight after quitting smoking

- Because smoking suppresses appetite, many of us worry about gaining weight when we quit smoking. You may be using it as an excuse not to quit. While it's true that many smokers gain weight in the first six months after quitting, the gain is relatively small, five pounds on average—and the weight gain gradually reduces with time. It's also worth remembering that gaining a few pounds for a few months won't harm your heart as much as smoking. However, gaining weight after quitting smoking is not a given.

- Because smoking dulls your senses of smell and taste, food will often seem more appealing when you quit. However, if you replace the oral enjoyment of smoking with unhealthy comfort foods, you may gain weight. As a result, rather than mindless, emotional eating, it's critical to discover other, healthier ways to deal with unpleasant feelings like stress, anxiety, or boredom.

- Take care of yourself. Learn new techniques to immediately comfort yourself instead of turning to cigarettes or food when you're upset, anxious, or depressed. For example, listen to cheerful music, play with a pet, or drink a cup of hot tea.

- Consume a variety of healthful foods. Consume a balanced diet of fruits, vegetables, and healthy fats. Sugary foods, sodas, fried foods, and convenience foods should all be avoided.

- Learn to eat mindfully. Emotional eating is usually unconscious and automatic. It's easy to devour a whole tub of ice cream while spacing out in front of the TV or staring at your phone. It's simpler to focus on how much you're eating and tune into your body and how you truly feel if you remove distractions while you eat. Are you still hungry, or are you eating for another reason?

- Make sure you get plenty of water. Drinking at least six to eight 8-ounce glasses of water will help you feel full and prevent eating when you aren't hungry. Water also assists in the elimination of toxins from the body. Take a stroll. It will not only help you burn calories and keep the weight off, but it will also help you cope with the stress and anguish that comes with quitting smoking.

- Snack on meals that don't make you feel bad. Sugar-free gum, carrot and celery sticks, sliced bell peppers, and jicama are all good options.

To assist you in quitting smoking, there is medication and treatment available.

There are a variety of ways that have proven to be effective in helping people quit smoking. While you may discover success with the first approach you try, it's more likely that you'll need to try various methods or a mix of treatments to find the ones that work best for you.

Medications

Smoking cessation drugs can help with withdrawal symptoms and cravings. However, they work best when used as part of a thorough quit-smoking program overseen by your doctor. Discuss your alternatives with your doctor to see if an anti-smoking drug is good for you. The following choices have been approved by the US Food and Drug Administration (FDA):

Nicotine replacement therapy. Nicotine replacement therapy uses nicotine substitutes such as nicotine gum, patch, lozenge, inhaler, or nasal spray to "replace" cigarettes. It helps to alleviate certain withdrawal symptoms by delivering small, consistent quantities of nicotine into your body without the tars and toxic chemicals found in cigarettes. In addition, this sort of treatment allows you to concentrate on breaking your psychological addiction while also learning new behaviors and coping skills.

Medication that does not include nicotine. Without the use of nicotine, these drugs help you quit smoking by lowering cravings and withdrawal symptoms. However, medications like bupropion (Zyban) and varenicline (Chantix, Champix) are only meant to be used briefly.

What you should know about electronic cigarettes (vaping)

While some people find that vaping helps them quit smoking, the FDA has not approved it as a smoking cessation technique. In recent news reports, Vaping has even been connected to severe lung disease, raising concerns about its safety. Here's what you should be aware of:

The FDA does not regulate e-cigarette products in the United States.

Vaping can be harmful "to youth, young adults, pregnant women, or individuals who do not currently use tobacco products," according to the FDA.

It's difficult to fully know what's in e-cigarettes.

Nicotine is present in the liquid used in some e-cigarettes, which has several harmful health impacts. It can cause high blood pressure and diabetes, and it's especially detrimental for children and teenagers' developing brains.

There is no evidence available on the long-term implications of vaping on one's health.

Federal and state officials advise that all vaping be avoided until additional information becomes available.

Alternative therapies

There are various alternatives to nicotine replacement treatment, vaping, or prescription drugs for quitting smoking. These are some of them:

Hypnosis - This is a popular alternative that has helped many smokers who are trying to quit. Forget what you've seen from stage hypnotists; hypnosis works by lulling you into a profound state of relaxation in which you're open to suggestions that will enhance your resolve to quit smoking and deepen your dislike for cigarettes.

Acupuncture is one of the oldest known medical procedures; it is believed to function by causing the body to relax by encouraging the production of endorphins (natural pain relievers). Acupuncture can assist manage smoking withdrawal symptoms as a smoking cessation therapy.

Behavioral Therapy - Nicotine addiction is linked to smoking's regular actions or routines. Learning new coping skills and changing bad habits are the main goals of behavior therapy.

Self-Help Books and Websites — Various self-help books and websites can help you quit smoking. Calculating monetary savings is a well-known example. Calculating how much money they will save has helped some people find the drive to quitIt's possible that it'll be enough to pay for a summer vacation.

Smokeless tobacco, sometimes known as spit tobacco, is not a healthy substitute for smoking.

Smokeless tobacco, also known as spit or chewing tobacco, is a dangerous substitute for cigarettes. This is because nicotine, the addictive ingredient found in cigarettes, is present in them. In fact, smokeless tobacco absorbs three to four times the amount of nicotine that a cigarette does.

What to do if you go off the wagon or relapse

Don't be too hard on yourself if you slip up and have a cigarette. Most individuals try to quit smoking several times before finally succeeding. Instead, learn from your mistake and transform your relapse into a rebound. Examine the events leading up to your resumption of smoking, identify the triggers or trouble spots you encountered, and devise a fresh stop-smoking strategy that removes them.

It's also critical to stress the distinction between a slip and a relapse. It doesn't imply you won't be able to quit if you start smoking again. You may either learn from your mistake and use it to motivate you to work harder in the future, or you can use it as an excuse to resume your smoking habit. However, you have the last say. A slip does not have to become a full-fledged relapse.

If you make a mistake, you are not a failure. However, that isn't to say you can't quit for good.

Allowing a slip to turn into a mudslide is not a good idea. The rest of the pack should be discarded. It's critical to return to a non-smoking lifestyle as soon as feasible.

Take a look back at your quit log and be proud of how long you could go without smoking.

Find the source of the problem. What prompted you to pick up a cigarette once more? Then, make a plan for how you'll handle the situation the next time it arises.

Take notes on what you've learned. What has been the most beneficial? What didn't go as planned?

Is there anything you're taking to help you quit smoking? If you start smoking again, contact your doctor. If you're smoking, you won't be able to take some medications.

Assisting a loved one in quitting smoking

It's crucial to remember that you can't force a friend or loved one to quit smoking; they must make their own decision. If they decide to stop smoking, you can offer support and encouragement while also attempting to alleviate the stress of quitting. Investigate the various therapy alternatives and discuss them with the smoker; however, never preach or pass judgment. You can also assist a smoker in overcoming cravings by engaging in other activities with them and having smoking replacements on standby, such as gum.

Don't make a loved one feel bad if they fall off the wagon or relapse. Instead, congratulate them on going without smokes for some time and urge them to try again. Your encouragement can make all the difference in your loved one's ability to finally stop the habit.

Assisting a teen in quitting smoking

Around the age of 11, most smokers take their first cigarette, and by the age of 14, many are addicted. In recent years, the usage of e-cigarettes (vaping) has also increased substantially. While the health effects of vaping aren't completely understood, the FDA advises that it's not safe for teenagers, and we do know that youths who vape are more likely to start smoking cigarettes. Parents may be concerned, but it's vital to recognize the unique problems and peer pressure that kids encounter while quitting smoking (or vaping). While the young smoker must decide to quit on their own, you can still do many things to help.

Parents of kids who smoke or vape should follow these guidelines.

• Find out why your kid is smoking or vaping; they may be trying to fit in with their peers or seeking your attention. Rather than issuing threats or deadlines, discuss what adjustments might be made in their lives to assist them in quitting smoking.

• If your youngster agrees to stop smoking, be patient and helpful during the process.

• Set a positive example by refusing to smoke. Smoking parents are more likely to have smoking children.

• Find out if your children's pals smoke or vape. Then, discuss how to refuse a cigarette or e-cigarette with them.

• Explain the risks to their health as well as the negative effects smoking can have on their looks (such as bad breath, discolored teeth, and nails).

• Create a no-smoking policy in your home. No one should be allowed to smoke or vape indoors at any time.

Chapter Eight

EXERCISE AWAY THE URGE OF SMOKING

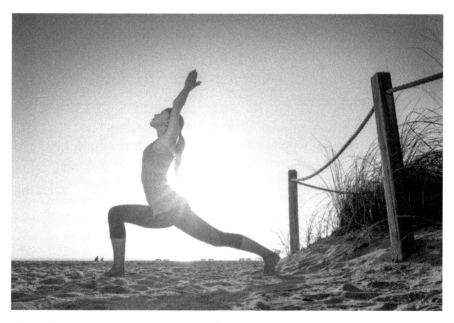

Working out is yet another fantastic approach for stress management, well-being, self-improvement, state of mind, and pretty much everything else.

Although there haven't been many studies on exercise and habit, researchers believe that working out is an excellent way to help you quit smoking for good.

This could be attributed to several factors.

1. Exercise aids in the normalization of your mental science and the smoothing out of your moods. As a result, you'll feel better and won't crave cigarettes nearly as much.

2. Exercise promotes deep relaxation. Because you're drawing oxygen deeply into your lungs, a piece of the hit you feel from a cigarette is due to this. Profound breathing is a good way to help yearnings fade away.

3. Exercise is beneficial to your health. It just focuses on your body a little, just enough to energize and strengthen it, but not enough to harm it (assuming you're doing the ideal exercise at the perfect power). This can help your body recover from the negative effects of smoking on your health.

4. Movement is a fun way to pass the time. Moving around is a good way to distract your mind and body from longings, and other withdrawal symptoms, especially early on in your quit smoking cycle.

5. Exercise provides you with a greater reward. Nicotine deceives the pleasure and reward centers of your brain, but exercise energizes them and replaces a fake award with a genuine one.

Apart from that, succeeding in one test increases your chances of succeeding in another. Thus, your goal of quitting smoking and your activity goals can complement each other.

Before beginning any sort of exercise, speak with your doctor. (While the specialist is unlikely to subdue you, they may have thoughts about what type of exercise is typically appropriate.) Also, talk to a local fitness center, a personal trainer, or a health coach about your goals and plan to achieve them.

Getting a Group Together: Collaborating

Smokers who are trying to stop can benefit by gathering support. Why not organize a meetup in your community or on Facebook or another social media platform? (According to a recent report, an informal online group that aided people in quitting smoking was recommended.)

Here Are Some Basic Tips For A Successful Quit Smoking Get-Together.

1. Advertise it in the appropriate places. Flyers on light poles, a local area noticeboard, a website, or distribution like a local paper or bulletin are examples of this. Consider where people who are trying to quit smoking will most likely notice it. You don't need a big marketing budget — if you tell a compelling tale, some local distributions will promote it for free.

2. Be unmistakable. If you're all nervous and try to figure out when people are free, what time suits them, where a good location could be, and how we could run it, it'll fail right away. Set a time frame, find an arrangement that works for you, and then advertise it. Give people something to think about that is upbeat.

3. Prepare a basic setup. Individuals will laze around awkwardly, staring at one another if nothing is planned. Everything will be overdone if everything is planned with a stopwatch. Make sure the nuts and bolts are covered: Everyone will speak (in a circle), you or another person will put on a brief show, and there should be some convivial time before or after with important prizes available.

4. Create a safe haven. The gathering should be a place where people can be open and honest about their feelings if they're having a good time (or if they're having a bad time), without feeling judged or slighted for what they're going through. Speaking honestly about how you feel is an excellent way to manage a wide range of emotions while also uniting a group.

5.When it's finished, it's done. It's a good idea to have a pre-determined timetable for when the group will meet — for example, every 14 days weeks, or every six or two months, depending on the type of people you're focusing on and how much time they have. If it's functioning well and people need to meet, you may usually choose to expand it. In any case, if no one else is coming or the meeting has met its purpose, let it end.

Returning to Your Former Self

Not everyone will tell you this since they don't want you to think about the possibility of "disappointment." Regardless, the vast majority of people who successfully quit smoking require several attempts (the normal is around 5). Obviously, the more and better your stop smoking assets are, the better your chances of outperforming the standard are.

I'd like to add three more points to that.

1. There is no such thing as a single cigarette. One is an excessive number, and 1,000 is insufficient. If you start smoking again after a while, especially two or three years, you will reawaken all of the parts of your mind that enjoy nicotine, and they will take over responsibility for you. That isn't required.

2. On the other hand, resuming smoking isn't a letdown. It's a form of critique. It's telling you that there's still something you need to

figure out to achieve your goal of quitting smoking. Make use of it, and don't be afraid to ask for more support from those who have previously assisted you.

3. If you start again, you must stop again. Consider it a new beginning. Plunge once more into your assets, possibly try a different plan, get some additional help, but somehow beat it.

What Is the Best Way to Begin Exercising?

To stay motivated, consider the following suggestions:

• Setting aside a regular time for exercise might be beneficial; choose a time that works for you.

• On most days of the week, aim for at least 30 minutes of moderate-intensity physical activity.

• Make fitness a priority and include it in your daily routine. If you don't have 30 minutes to spare, you can workout in 10-minute increments.

• Make sure you choose activities that you are comfortable with. Begin slowly and gradually increase the frequency and intensity of your workouts.

• Signing up for a class or arranging to work out with someone else may make it easier to stick to your goals.

Suggestions for Exercise

You don't have to put yourself through a workout like a kickboxing the first time you go. It's fine to start slowly:

One strategy to increase your physical activity is to go for a walk. Take a walk during your lunch break or after supper with a coworker, friend, or family member. Make sure to find non-smoking friends! Increase the length and speed of your walks gradually.

Consider other activities you might love, such as riding, swimming, dance, or yoga – almost any sport will assist.

Housework and gardening are also good ways to get some exercise. There's also the matter of cleaning out the garage. Playing music that you appreciate will assist you in increasing your pace.

Plan physical activity-based family activities or social gatherings, such as hiking, volleyball, or a trip to the beach.

<u>When a Craving Strikes, Exercising at Work</u>

You're at work, and the want to smoke is driving you insane. But, in your job clothing, what kind of workout can you do? Plenty.

- Deep knee bends are a good thing to do.
- Take a few steps up and down a flight of stairs.
- Alternate between relaxing and tensing your muscles while sitting at your workstation.
- Close your office door or go somewhere quiet to do some push-ups. If you don't want to go down on the floor, try standing push-ups against a wall.

<u>Maintaining Your Exercise Routine</u>

When smokers engage in physical exertion, they frequently experience shortness of breath. However, once you've quit, you'll undoubtedly realize that exercising is becoming simpler. This is because quitting smoking improves your lung function.

Some people enjoy exercising, while others find it challenging to maintain a consistent fitness practice. After a while, boredom can set in. Changing up your regimen or type of exercise, on the other hand, can be beneficial. Consider enrolling in a fitness class or learning a new activity. Set a goal for yourself, such as running a race or competing in a tournament. The competitive challenge might be exactly what you're looking for.

Chapter Nine

ROADMAP DEFINITION

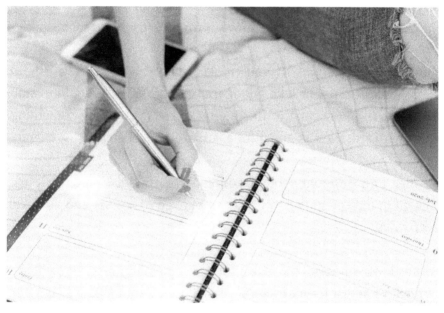

S et a deadline for quitting. Choose a day when you will stop smoking. Make a note of it on your calendar and inform loved ones (if they are aware) that you will be stopping on that day. Consider the day as a dividing line between you as a smoker and the new, improved nonsmoker you'll become.

Throw away your cigarettes – all of them — out the window. Individuals will be unable to quit smoking if cigarettes are available to tempt them. So get rid of everything, including ashtrays, lighters, and even the emergency pack you hid.

All of your clothes should be washed. Wash all of your clothes and get your jackets or sweaters dry-cleaned to get rid of the cigarette odor as much as possible. If you smoked in your car, make sure to clean it up as well.

Take into account your personal triggers. You're probably aware of the times when you'll smoke in general, such as after dinners, while you're at a close friend's house while drinking espresso, or when driving. Something that makes you feel compelled to smoke is a trigger. When you've figured out your triggers, try these suggestions:

•break the connections. If you smoke while driving, seek a ride to class, walk to class, or take public transportation for a month to stop the habit. If you normally smoke after dinners, try doing something new afterward, such as going for a stroll or conversing with a friend.

•change to a different spot. If you and your buddies frequently eat takeout in the car so that you may smoke, go to a diner and evaluate everything.

•Instead of smokes, try substituting something else. It will be difficult to adjust to not holding something or not having a cigarette in your mouth in general. If you have this problem, keep carrot sticks, sugar-free gum, mints, toothpicks, and confections on hand.

How to Deal With Withdrawal

Expect some physical manifestations. If you quit using nicotine and your body becomes addicted to it, you may experience withdrawal symptoms. Withdrawal symptoms might include:

•headaches, migraines, or stomachaches

•nervousness, crabbiness, or a sense of pessimism

•energy deficiency

•a painful throat or a dry mouth

•the desire to eat

The nicotine withdrawal need will pass, so exercise restraint. Make a conscious effort to avoid quitting and sneaking a cigarette, as you'll have to deal with the withdrawal for a longer period.

Maintain your involvement. Several people believe that stopping on a Monday when they have school or work is the best way to keep them engaged. The more active you get, the less likely you are to need smokes. Maintaining agility is also a nice distraction, and it aids in keeping your weight down and your energy up.

Stop in small steps. A few organizations have discovered that gradually reducing the number of cigarettes they consume each day is an effective way to quit. This technique, however, does not work for everyone. You may believe that going "clean and simple" and quitting smoking at the same time is the best option for you.

If you really want to quit smoking, look into using a nicotine substitute. If none of these methods work, talk to your primary care physician about nicotine replacement gums, patches, inhalers, or nasal sprays. Showers and inhalers are only available through medication, and you should contact your primary care physician before buying the fix and gum over the counter. In addition, various drugs have unanticipated effects (for instance, the fix is not difficult to utilize, yet different medicines offer a quicker kick of nicotine).

Again, your primary health care provider can help you to find the optimum solution for you.

Mistakes occur

Don't give up if you make a mistake! Significant shifts can have phony beginnings. If you're like most people, you may be able to stop for a long time, even months, and then suddenly have a strong desire that makes you feel compelled to give in. Alternatively, you may find yourself in one of your trigger situations and succumb to enticement.

If you make a mistake, it doesn't mean you've failed. It simply means you're a person. So here are three methods for refocusing:

1. Consider your mistake as a single one. Then, pay attention to when and why it happened before moving on.

2. Did one cigarette turn you into a regular smoker? Almost certainly not. It happened slowly and gradually over time. Remember that one cigarette did not make you a smoker in the first place and that smoking one (or even a few) after you quit will not make you a smoker again.

3. Remind yourself why you quit and how well you've done — or have someone from your support group, family, or friends do it for you.

Give yourself a prize. It's not easy to quit smoking. So give yourself a well-deserved reward! Set aside the money you would normally spend on smokes. Give yourself a treat when you've gone tobacco-free for seven, fourteen, or a month. It may be a gift card, a movie, or some new clothes. Every year that there isn't any smoke, it's time to celebrate once more. You earned it.

Chapter Ten

ADDITIONAL TIPS AND METHODS

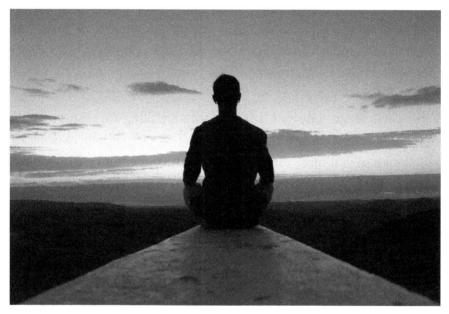

1. All things considered, if you're trying to quit smoking, give chewing gum a try. In general, if you want to get rid of a bad habit, you should replace it with a more reliable one. Gum chewing allows you to use your mouth and jaw in some of the same ways that smoking does. It's a good way to keep yourself occupied when you're attempting to stop.

2. Some people believe they can quit smoking by switching to a different product, such as chewing tobacco. This isn't a good idea because chewing tobacco has more nicotine than a cigarette. You may end up swapping one urge for another. If you genuinely need something to help you stop, try nicotine gums, all other things being equal. The gums can be gradually tightened. Unfortunately, they don't usually sell more sensitive biting tobacco types dynamically.

3. If you're trying to quit smoking, make sure you get plenty of rest. Many people discover that they are more likely to crave cigarettes if they stay up late. Furthermore, you will be isolated from everyone else late in the evening, increasing your desire to smoke. Getting plenty of sleep will not only cut down on the amount of time you spend daydreaming about cigarettes, but it will also help your body cope with nicotine withdrawal.

4. Be clear about why you need to stop smoking to keep yourself motivated to quit. While there are countless compelling reasons to quit smoking, you must focus on your own unique set of compelling reasons. When you're tempted, remind yourself of how much you need to improve your health, lay aside money, or set a good example for your children.

5. Discuss professionally recommended medications with your primary care physician. Consider using medications prescribed by your doctor to help with nicotine withdrawal symptoms. Certain medications can aid reduce yearnings by influencing the chemical equilibrium in your cerebrum. There are also sedates that can help with vexing withdrawal symptoms like inability to think or melancholy.

6. If you're quitting smoking, you'll need to figure out how to manage your stress. When smoking is no longer an option, turn to healthier alternatives like kneading, long walks in your favorite park,

listening to relaxing music, or contemplation. Find something you can do that gives you immediate gratification, so you're less tempted to turn to smoke when things become tough.

7. Changing the brand of cigarettes you smoke can assist you in quitting. Consider smoking a brand that you dislike. Try not to smoke more than once a day or in a different way. This will get you started on your journey to quit smoking.

8. Many smokers have distinct triggers that cause them to crave a cigarette suddenly, like being focused, finishing a meal, or being in a specific location. If at all possible, keep away from these triggers when attempting to stop. If you can't stay away from them, come up with a technique to distract yourself from the urge to smoke.

9. Discover interesting facts about how quitting smoking will benefit your health. There are countless studies out there that show how significantly lower your chances of developing illnesses are if you don't smoke. Also, find out how soon you might expect to notice other minor benefits such as better breathing and a better sense of taste.

10. Keep a journal of each time you smoke a cigarette and why you did so. This journal will help you figure out what makes you want to smoke. It could be the first-morning cigarette or the need to smoke after supper for others. For others, it could very well be a source of stress. Identifying your triggers will aid you in devising a strategy to combat them.

11. To make quitting smoking appear more straightforward, quantify the negative aspects of your smoking proclivity. Sort out how often you smoke, how many cigarettes you consume every day, and how much it costs you to smoke that many cigarettes on a daily, monthly,

and yearly basis. You'll be able to see exactly how much you've progressed each time you cut back a little.

12. It will be easier to resist allurement if you can get rid of objects that remind you of smoking. So you should get rid of ashtrays and cigarette lighters, among other things. To get rid of smoke odors in your home, clean it and wash your clothes. Because you're removing expected triggers, taking these steps may reduce your desire to light a cigarette.

13. Remind yourself of how messy cigarettes are. This will help you focus on stopping because you will be thinking about how messy they are. For example, avoid emptying ashtrays so you can see how much you've smoked and the foul odor it leaves behind. As an addition, you might also want to try filling a jar with the butts and remnants.

14. Begin exercising! If you're active, it can help with symptoms of withdrawal and nicotine cravings. Then, instead of going for a cigarette, get out of your chair and work out or go for a walk. This can greatly assist you in quitting smoking and is also an excellent way to improve your physical well-being.

15. Positive reasoning has a significant impact on quitting smoking. If you consider each day without smoking to be a victory in and of itself, you will be more willing to overcome temptations. In addition, by keeping track of small goals, you may maintain your confidence and, hopefully, overcome your proclivity for greatness!

16. You must follow a healthy dietary plan. Avoid quitting smoking and begin an eating plan at the same time. Instead, maintain a healthy, well-balanced dietary routine. If you smoke, vegetables and natural products can be harmful.

If you smoke, you'll notice a difference in flavor. Eating these foods while you don't smoke will benefit your health and help you avoid those harmful smokes.

17. If you want to quit smoking, the word "No" is for you. You must deny yourself the ability to say "Yes" to a cigarette every time you are lured. If your only answer is "No," you'll quickly realize that you can't give in to a craving. There will be no smoking if there are no cigarettes.

18. Reward yourself if you're succeeding in your smoking cessation efforts. When you've cut back, treat yourself to a good back rub, a pedicure, or a great new dress, and then do something different when you've entirely stopped. You need to be able to anticipate rewards like this, as they can help you stay motivated.

19. Take care of nicotine withdrawal symptoms. Nicotine withdrawal might make you feel restless, frustrated, or discouraged after you stop smoking. It's usually quite simple to revert to your former habits. Nicotine replacement therapy can help to alleviate these adverse effects. Whether as gum, a fix, or a capsule, using one of them will almost certainly double your chances of success.

20. Make sure you don't feel obligated to give up any aspect of your life because you've quit smoking. As an ex-smoker, you are free to do whatever you want. Who knows, you might even be able to accomplish your number one item a little bit better.

21. If you're a smoker who lights up more in social situations, make plans to avoid joining your friends for a cigarette when you're out. If your dining friends walk outside to smoke, stay at the table. Find a non-smoker to chat with if you're at a gathering where people are smoking. It will be easier for you to quit smoking to figure out how to avoid social situations with smokers.

22. When you want to quit smoking, the most important thing you can do is make that fundamental commitment to change. Rather than setting a deadline that you can keep pushing back, quit now. Simply stop smoking and promise yourself that you will never do so again. Although this technique is time-consuming, the benefits are enormous. In addition, the strategy is the most effective in the long run.

23. Write down why you're quitting early and keep the list handy. When you have a craving, look through your list for ideas. Understanding why quitting is important to you early on will help you stay focused in those moments of failure, and it may even help you get back into the swing of things if you make a mistake.

24. A nicotine withdrawal medicine does not have to contain nicotine. While the facts show that you can find a substitute source of nicotine and reduce your nicotine levels, you might just try a doctor-prescribed medication that meets your nicotine needs. Consult your doctor about a prescription that could help you achieve your goals.

25. Get your feet moving. Actual work is excellent for reducing nicotine cravings and easing certain withdrawal symptoms. So when you're craving a cigarette, all things considered, go for a run.

Even light activity might be beneficial, such as removing weeds in the nursery or taking a relaxing walk. Furthermore, the added activity will burn more calories and help you avoid weight gain when you quit smoking.

26. All things considered, you can replace your smoking proclivity with a positive adaptive proclivity. This entails looking deep inside yourself and understanding your tendencies. For example, if you smoke when you're nervous, think about how you can distribute the

negative energy, all things being equal. Some people find comfort in mindful and deep breathing exercises; however, you can experiment with various techniques to find one that works for you.

27. If you want to quit smoking, don't buy cigarettes. It goes without saying that it will be much more difficult to smoke if you don't have any cigarettes with you. So discard whatever smokes you currently own and promise yourself that you will not acquire any more.

28. To make quitting smoking appear more straightforward, convert the unfavorable aspects of your smoking proclivity into statistics. Sort out how often you smoke, how many cigarettes you consume every day, and how much it costs you to smoke that many cigarettes on a daily, monthly, and yearly basis. Each time you cut back a little, you'll be able to see just how far you've come.

29. Make every effort to avoid starting to smoke without first establishing an arrangement. Cigarettes have most likely controlled your life for a long time. A life without cigarettes will necessitate alterations in your daily routine. Choosing what to do about cravings, avoiding triggers, and establishing a quit date are all essential components of a successful quit plan.

30. Exercise can aid in the cessation of smoking. After you exercise, your brain releases endorphins, which improve your mood. Exercising is also a fantastic way to break up with your desires. Exercise will also assist your digestion in compensating for the impact it gets when you stop smoking, reducing the likelihood of weight gain.

31. Eat veggies, organic food, seeds, and nuts while you are quitting smoking. For various reasons, sticking to a consistent, well-balanced diet of common foods can be beneficial. To begin, you may usually replace smoking movements by keeping your lips and hands busy.

Additionally, your chances of gaining weight during this time of quitting are reduced. Nutritional pills and other supplements can also help you feel better when you're going through withdrawals.

32. If you're attempting to quit smoking, "pure and simple" quitting is a bad idea. Stopping smoking without a strategy to help with nicotine withdrawal is problematic. Because nicotine is a habit-forming substance, it's easy to relapse if you don't have some support while quitting. When you're ready to quit smoking, it's best to use smoking cessation medicine or some other type of treatment.

33. Keep crunchy foods like carrots or celery close by to keep your hands and mouth engaged when trying to quit smoking. These low-calorie snacks will not only keep you satisfied but will also help you lose weight.

On the other hand, keeping your hands occupied will keep your blood sugar stable and prevent you from eating other fatty foods, leading to weight gain.

34. Although revulsion therapies have received a lot of criticism recently, they do work in some instances to help you quit smoking. They don't have to be extravagant, and you don't have to hire a professional to use repugnance procedures. Instead, try simple things like saturating your #1 sweater with the cigarette smoke from the last one you smoked. Then, after not smoking for a while, go after it; you'll be surprised at the foul odor you've been subjecting yourself and others to regularly.

35. You must speak with a professional before quitting smoking. This person can offer you advice on the best ways to stop. In addition, the individual may be able to provide you with additional assistance during your journey. Both of these factors greatly increase your chances of making a great stop.

36. Your friends and family rely on you to quit smoking for their health. Smoking is harmful to you and anybody around you who breathes in secondhand smoke, and it can even cause sickness. If you stop smoking, you are removing used smoke from the lives of your friends and family. When you stop smoking, not only will you feel better, but your friends and family will feel better as well.

37. If you want to improve your chances of quitting smoking for good, don't combine your efforts to quit with another goal, such as weight loss. You've already got enough stress and desires to deal with just trying to quit smoking. If you try to wean yourself from something else simultaneously, you'll probably fail at both.

38. As you begin your journey to a smoke-free lifestyle, set a succession of remunerations as you reach specific goals. Make a list of the rewards you'll give yourself for quitting smoking for one day, seven days, a month, and so on. Put this list on your cooler and look at it every day before going to work or school. This could very well help you stay motivated during times of adversity.

39. Make it clear to yourself that you will not smoke every day. When you first wake up in the morning, try telling yourself that you won't smoke a single cigarette. Reaffirming this goal in your mind every morning will keep you on track to successful smoking cessation.

40. Invest the time and money you save by quitting smoking in working out. Exercise releases mood-boosting endorphins, and physical labor will keep you occupied and distracted from your desires. Exercise can also assist you in avoiding gaining weight as a result of the changes in your digestion that nicotine withdrawal might bring about.

Chapter Eleven

COMMON PROBLEMS IN QUITTING SMOKING

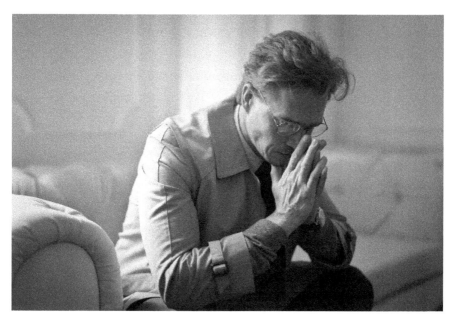

A fter you've quit smoking, here are some solutions to some of the most common problems you'll face.

People give up and go back to smoking because they are in excruciating pain and don't know how to handle their problems quickly. Here are a few pointers to help you get through the frequent challenges that arise when you quit smoking as painlessly as possible.

Anger, anxiety, irritability, and mood swings.

"Before you will be set free, the truth will annoy you." Gloria Steinem When you stop smoking, you may turn into a rage-filled jerk. Alternatively, it could be a teary, emotional disaster. This is due in part to chemical changes in the brain and in part to the fact that you have utilized smoking to cope with your emotions. When you lose your coping technique, your feelings may become overwhelming and seem much more strong. This is inconvenient and aggravating for both you and those around you.

One of the most common reasons smokers postpone, delay, or abandon their attempts to quit smoking is because of these extreme mood swings. Your heightened anger and frustration impacts not only you but also those with whom you spend time. We utilize the increase in negative feelings as an excuse to keep smoking.

The truth is that you didn't abandon your decision to quit smoking because of your hostility, impatience, or short temper; it was because you didn't have the tools and resources to effectively handle this component of the process. Deep down, dealing with transient anger and moodiness isn't a good enough cause to keep smoking.

Walking on eggshells while going through withdrawals is not something the world owes you. You can't expect others to change their behavior to make up for your bad mood. If everyone around you has to cater to your grumpiness for you not to behave insanely, you're going to be fairly lonely in the end.

You may eventually discover that part of the anger you're experiencing isn't totally related to quitting smoking. Whatever the source of the anger, it must be addressed in a way that avoids relapsing into unhealthy, self-destructive addictions that are merely concealing the pain you aren't dealing with. In some circumstances, our rage is simply a repressed childhood memory. In the same way, one of our carers.

We are sometimes aware of what is giving us pain, and other times we are aware that we are unhappy but don't know why. You can bury the sorrow by hiding it. The trouble is that pain isn't natural, and it won't go away by pretending it isn't there, so we turn to cigarettes, alcohol, food, and narcotics to alleviate our discomfort.

Getting in touch with your sorrow and bad childhood programs and letting them go will help you let go of your desire to numb yourself with harmful substances. Our mind and body are inextricably linked. We have more control over our behavior, body, and lives if we know what influences us and how to best deal with it.

Several techniques can assist you in reaching that point of calm and avoiding the same destructive cycles. Hypnotherapy, Counseling, Cognitive Behavioral Therapy (CBT), Psychotherapy, Neuro-Linguistic Programming (NLP), Meditation, Eye Patch Therapy, Tapping (EFT), Deep Breathing, and Visualization are just a few of the methods that can help us change our beliefs and behaviors.

A smoker can become a peaceful, happy ex-smoker who deals with their emotions even more efficiently than they did before by devising effective techniques to control the anger, anxiety, and irritation that is so prevalent while quitting smoking.

Anger and Irritability: What You Need to Know

We can come across things that irritate us daily. Common causes include feelings of:

- Frustration
- Feeling like you're being scrutinized or criticized

- feeling bothered or harassed

- Injustice, whether genuine or perceived.

- Feeling left out or like your needs aren't being met

- Requests that we do not want to fulfill or that we consider are unjust

- Threats against the people, objects, or concepts we care about

A lot of how we behave is influenced by our upbringing and how the people in our lives reacted to stress. Anger is elicited in various persons for various reasons and in various ways. Something that annoys you slightly may enrage someone else completely. Anger is incredibly personal, yet the more you become aware of it, the more you realize that how you respond to it is entirely up to you.

So, what are some ways to deal with the feelings of rage, anxiety, frustration, and irritability that come with quitting smoking and life in general?

Here are some strategies that I have personally discovered to be the most effective.

- Name It To Tame It

- The 4 + 4 + 8 Breat

- Radical Acceptance

- H.A.L.T

- Tapping Guided Relaxation/ Hypnosis

Breathing a few deep breaths and counting to 10 are other excellent ways for dealing with anger as it arises, in addition to taking a timeout. Boxing, punching a punching bag, yoga, and even building a pile of pillows and hitting them with a bat are all good ways to let out pent-up rage.

Name it to tame it

Dan Siegel, a psychologist, coined the phrase "name it to tame it." His research has shown that naming our emotions helps calm down our brain's fear center while also activating the prefrontal cortex, which helps us manage our behavior.

"When you take time for your feelings, you become less stressed, and you can think more clearly and creatively, making it easier to develop constructive solutions," adds Dr. Dean Ornish. We can't change what we don't understand. Avoiding, suppressing, or lashing out at our feelings does not make them go away or lessen their influence on us. Identifying and naming our emotions allows us to pause and take a step back, allowing us to make healthy decisions about dealing with them.

Emotions, in my opinion, are a sort of energy that yearns to be expressed. E-motions- must be able to move. Even the most turbulent emotions can be managed and controlled by just stating what you're experiencing. You can help shift and release your emotions by naming them aloud. Due to this reason, they are less likely to spew at the expense of others.

It's fine to have emotions and feelings. It's quite normal to get angry, wounded, irritated, exasperated, or upset. However, it's not acceptable to strike out improperly against those who don't deserve it. Being angry or unhappy was my largest trigger for relapsing with smoking. I used to smoke to cope with my feelings, but I wasn't actually dealing with them. I was only using nicotine to numb them.

Exercise: Name It To Tame It

This practice raises your awareness by identifying the type of emotion you're experiencing and assisting you in releasing it. It might also help you figure out if there's a pattern from the past.

Try saying or writing something like this:

I'm feeling_____.

I am feeling this way because _____.

I felt this way before when_____.

_____ (yourself or someone close to you) used to react this way when I was younger when_____happened.

Feel the emotions and where they are located in your body. Imagine drawing the emotions into your lungs like black smoke and then exhaling the black smoke/emotions as you inhale. With each breath, let go of any bad emotions.

Radical Acceptance

"Truth is similar to poetry. And the vast majority of people despise poetry." The Big Short Film

Expectations, resistance to change, and a refusal to accept what is happening now cause a lot of our stress. Your mind is a fear-based system that is concerned mainly with survival in the past and future. It is always analyzing, comparing, judging, and nagging you about what you or others should do to improve, be accepted, be happier, or be more successful.

Your mind can be a harsh critic of you or what's going on in your life right now. It enjoys talking about your and other people's flaws, as well as how useless, stupid, unattractive, or unworthy you or they are. The trouble is that a lot of what your mind thinks about isn't true. So unless you realize that your mind tells you many lies, you will trust what it says.

The majority of individuals fight what is going on in their life, as though things should be different. This never-ending struggle of resistance is stressful and pointless. Almost all of our feelings of rage, disappointment, frustration, anguish, and discontent stem from our opposition to or disagreement with some current aspect of our lives.

Acceptance does not imply that you should lie down and play dead, that you should tolerate an abusive environment, or that you should become complacent. On the contrary, accepting reality gives you power. Accepting the way people and events right now give you control and the ability to alter what you can. It can be frightening when something terrible occurs, but years later, we can nearly always look back and see what good came from it. The accidents, job losses, and the end of a relationship that prompted us to change our lives for the better are examples of how such "traumas" put us on a path we would not have taken otherwise.

"This is perfect, this is what I want" is an excellent mantra to have to assist us in getting through a difficult scenario.

Every cell in your body may be screaming, "THIS IS NOT PERFECT!" at the time. THIS IS NOT WHAT I AM LOOKING FOR!" Looking at life from this perspective, on the other hand, allows you to be empowered and adaptable to change rather than a victim of it.

Consider times when something happened that caused you many worries, but then the situation changed for the better. For example, you may lose your job and then find a new one that is much more suited to you, or you may stop a relationship and then meet someone you are much happier with. When you quit smoking, you will experience discomfort and have to cope with cravings in the short term, but there will be many long-term benefits.

More tools to help you stay calm

H.A.L.T. (High-Altitude Long-Term Training) –ask yourself if you're hungry, angry, lonely, or tired? Stopping for a moment and becoming aware of how you're feeling and what you require at the time might sometimes help you change your mood. Remember that the irritability that comes with quitting smoking will pass and that it is only temporary. We tend to keep pushing without taking care of ourselves, putting other people's demands ahead of our own, until we snap. When I start to feel this way, I know the best thing I can do is lie down for a short period - even if it's only 15 minutes.

Accept Your Feelings - Many of us, especially women, have been taught that getting angry is not okay. That we should grin and act as if everything is fine, even if it isn't. We hide our rage behind a tight-lipped smile when we're raging on the inside. Rather than being honest about how we feel and what we're furious about, many of us choose to be passive-aggressive.

The trouble is that people can see right through what you're hiding on the inside, so you're only deceiving yourself. It's much healthier to just say it out loud but in a calm and vulnerable manner. It's difficult to dispute with someone who expresses their thoughts calmly and clearly, without blaming others and accepting full responsibility for their emotions.

Keep in mind that practically everything is temporary, and whatever you're feeling right now will change, even if it doesn't feel like it. You have to manage your emotions, yet nicotine withdrawal tends to transform us into aggressive, thoughtless jerks. Your actions impact those who have nothing to do with your anger. Yes, it's all too easy to give in to your rage and vent it on someone close to you. But it's up to you to recognize when this will happen and prevent yourself from exploding in rage and embarrassing yourself.

Sometimes it's just too much, and before we realize it, we're screaming at some poor high school student serving us at the movie theater because they forgot to butter our popcorn. In this situation, the greatest thing you can do is accept responsibility. "Please accept my heartfelt apologies. I recently quit smoking. I'm not like this usually, and you didn't deserve it. Please accept my apologies." Then you cross your fingers that he doesn't go away with your popcorn and add his own special sauce. Every action has a reciprocal and opposing response; they will undoubtedly do the same if you scream and holler at someone. What you send out into the world will come back to haunt you. This is a universal law that I have always believed to be true.

Constipation

Constipation is caused by a temporary decrease in bowel motions as your body adjusts to not having nicotine to stimulate it when you stop smoking. It usually lasts a couple of weeks.

You can relieve constipation by doing the following:

Your liver and bowel are stimulated to release toxins when you drink hot water with fresh lemon juice first thing in the morning. If you're truly stuck, add a spoonful of olive oil. (If you don't take the olive oil on an empty stomach, it won't work.)

Take walks, do yoga, or engage in any other form of physical activity.

Make sure you get lots of water (at least 6-8 glasses daily). According to a new study, consuming 16 ounces of water before meals can result in a weight loss of 4.3 kg (9 pounds) over 12 weeks. This method is ideal for avoiding the weight gain after stopping smoking.

Fiber (fruits, vegetables, oats, flaxseeds, chia seeds, psyllium husks) serves as an internal broom, cleaning toxins out of your system. Fiber can also aid with weight loss and hormone imbalances by flushing out extra estrogens.

Take a large glass of water with one tablespoon of psyllium husks (the main ingredient in Metamucil). After that, drink another glass of water to ensure that the psyllium doesn't absorb too much water as it goes through your digestive system. You can gradually increase your dosage to three times each day. Make sure you consume it immediately; otherwise, it will taste like muck.

Get some bentonite clay, liquid, or powder, and mix a teaspoon with the psyllium husks and water if you want to go all out. The combo of bentonite clay and psyllium husks is one of the most potent detoxes.

Warning: psyllium husks and bentonite clay can make your feces seem like black seaweed. The mixture is pulling off the mucoid plaque on your intestinal walls.

The mucoid plaque and how it affects you

Your intestines produce mucus as a self-defense mechanism. Mucus builds up over time due to poor eating habits and a sluggish colon, resulting in a black, sticky, and rubbery-textured substance. The mucoid plaque is a seaweed-like substance that contains mucus, undigested food, feces, parasites, bacteria, and toxins. Ewww!

Finally, if you do become constipated, MagO7 is a go-to supplement. This is not a laxative, but it does help remove old matter by bringing oxygen into the body. Mag O7 Oxygen Cleanse breaks down and removes old junk, as well as hazardous bacteria in your gut, while the magnesium in it softens intestinal buildup and removes unnecessary waste.

Headaches and dizziness

You may suffer dizziness and headaches when your body begins to receive more oxygen. The body receives extra oxygen through the blood, causing what appears to be hyperventilation. The dilating blood vessels in your head contribute to the headaches. When you stop drinking coffee after a long period, you may experience the same symptoms.

Tips for coping with dizziness and headaches include:

- Stretch and take a few calm, deep breaths (like yawning).
- Ice packs, cold gel packs, or a damp cloth placed on the forehead or wrapped around the back of the neck (frozen for ten minutes for a DIY ice pack) can help relieve headaches.
- Apply ice packs to your head while bathing in a warm bath with Epsom salts, baking soda, and a few drops of lavender essential oil.
- Rub a few drops of lavender or peppermint oil on your temples and forehead. To assist ease pain and tension, mix two to three drops of lavender or peppermint oil with coconut or massage oil and rub it into the shoulders, back of neck, forehead, and temples.
- Seek medical help if the headaches are severe or do not go away. As instructed, take pain relievers such as Tylenol, Paracetamol, or Excedrin. During the day, a painkiller with caffeine, such as Excedrin, is beneficial because it helps to

constrict the blood vessels that are partially responsible for the headache. This isn't ideal, but it's still better than smoking. Remember that this headache is produced by enhanced circulation and increased blood flow to your brain. Increased blood flow is beneficial to your health, cognitive function, and the appearance of your skin. Keep in mind that the headaches will subside after the first week.

Excessive Hunger

When you initially quit smoking, your blood sugar levels may plummet. Low blood sugar is often to blame for many of the negative symptoms reported during the first week. This blood sugar dip is often the origin of symptoms like dizziness, headaches, lack of focus, and the voracious hunger many people experience after quitting smoking. Sugar is the brain's preferred fuel, and when it's depleted, your brain can't function at its best.

The lack of the stimulating impact of nicotine on your blood sugar is the cause of your low blood sugar after stopping smoking. Cigarettes induce the liver to release sugar and fat reserves. This is one of the ways smoking works as an appetite suppressant and affects the satiety regions of your brain in the hypothalamus. Nicotine works faster than food when it comes to blood sugar levels.

When you eat to elevate blood sugar levels, it might take up to 20 minutes for the food to be absorbed and released into the bloodstream, which then powers the brain. Cigarettes cause the body to discharge its sugar stores in seconds, not 20 minutes. When you smoke regularly, your body doesn't have to release as much sugar on its own since you're utilizing nicotine to do it for you.

This is why, after quitting smoking, people tend to binge eat. They reduce blood sugar and desire to eat something sweet to make themselves feel better. On the other hand, they continue to feel bad long after eating their meal. It just takes a few minutes to eat, but it takes an average of 20 minutes for your blood sugar to rise following the initial swallow.

You eat a little extra because you don't feel any better right away. Some people will continue to eat until their blood sugar levels stabilize and they begin to feel better. This is one of the reasons why we continue to eat even when we are full. Your body will adjust and begin to release glucose/ sugar as needed by the third or fourth day, but you won't have the regular amounts of nicotine to give you a boost without eating.

Weight

To help balance your blood sugar, eat protein with every meal and snack on fruit if you feel your blood sugar crashing the first few days after quitting smoking. If your blood sugar is dangerously low, drink unsweetened fruit juices such as apple, blueberry, cranberry, orange, grape, and pomegranate. It's easier to dilute it by mixing it with soda water and ice. This should no longer be essential after the fourth day, as your body will begin to release sugar stores as it did previously.

To help keep your blood sugar in check, consume slow-release complex carbs like berries, melons, cherries, apples, plums, pears, sweet potatoes, yams, or quinoa. Eat fast-release carbs within 30 minutes of finishing a resistance-training activity to get the most effect. Changing your eating habits to one that is more consistent may be beneficial. This doesn't imply you should eat more, but it may be beneficial to redistribute your food into smaller, more regular meals so that your blood sugar remains stable throughout the day.

If you're still experiencing symptoms of low blood sugar after day five, it might be time to seek nutritional counsel from a professional.

Now is an excellent time to concentrate on your health and fitness. You'll have more energy and time to develop better habits and a healthier body. Remember that the average smoker smokes for one hour every day. This time is dedicated to a habit you've developed. Imagine how great you'd feel and look if you made it a practice to spend an hour each day focusing on eating well and exercising.

We are, in fact, the sum of our habits. Learned behaviors that are done over and over are referred to as habits. The majority of people are unaware of their habits and do not make an effort to change them for the better. This is unfortunate because your habits have the power to make or ruin you.

Avoiding non-organic white carbohydrates is a smart place to start when it comes to balancing blood sugar levels. All bread, cereal, spaghetti, tortillas, and fried items with a crumb coating should be avoided.

One reason to avoid white processed meals is chlorine dioxide, which is one of the chemicals used to bleach food long after it has become brown. When chlorine dioxide reacts with wheat protein, it produces alloxan, a toxin that attacks the pancreas and reduces its ability to make insulin.

Researchers are well aware of this link, and they employ alloxan to cause diabetes in experimental rats. Did you notice that? It's used to induce diabetes! If you eat anything white or "enriched," this is terrible news. White flour is used as a foundation in most whole wheat bread.

Most wheat, buckwheat, canola, corn, flax, lentils, oats, peas, soy, rye, potatoes, sugar beets, and sunflower crops are now sprayed with a weed killer (glyphosate) before harvest.

Glyphosate manufacturers argue that it is safe for humans and animals because what it kills in plants isn't present in mammals. However, in our microbes, glyphosate kills in plants are present, which is critical to understanding how it causes widespread systemic harm in humans and animals.

Bacteria outnumber cells in your body by a factor of ten. There are ten different types of microorganisms for every cell in your body, and they are all negatively affected by glyphosate. Our bacteria's health and life cycle are thought to be severely disrupted by glyphosate. Worse, glyphosate targets the beneficial bacteria first, allowing diseases to overgrow and take control.

According to scientists, our gut bacteria may be one of the most important aspects of keeping a healthy weight and overall health. So the moral of the tale is if you don't want to gain weight, avoid white foods and try to eat organic wherever possible.

Insomnia

Insomnia is a condition that almost everyone experiences at some point in their lives. Sleep deprivation is used as a kind of torture because it will irritate you. When you stop smoking, insomnia is a typical side effect. Here are some suggestions for dealing with it.

1. Reduce or eliminate your caffeine intake. Caffeine is a stimulant that everyone is aware of, but did you know that smokers metabolize caffeine at twice the rate of non-smokers? That implies it will leave your system more quickly. As a result, if you don't smoke, you're more sensitive to caffeine and are more likely to feel agitated and restless from a dose you could previously manage well. Replace your coffee with green tea or cut your caffeine intake in half.

2. At least an hour before bedtime, turn off all electronics.

The blue light emitted by most electronic devices reduces your natural melatonin production. As a result, you will be less sleepy at night. I get it; we're all addicted to our screens. Unfortunately, our biology has not kept up with our technological obsession.

3. At night, take a warm bath or shower.

Your body temperature drops naturally at night, starting two hours before you go to bed and peaking at 4 a.m. or at 5:00 a.m. When you take a bath and raise your temperature by a degree or two, the decrease in temperature that follows is more likely to put you into a deep slumber sooner. A shower isn't as effective as a bath, but it can assist.

One to two hours before bedtime, soak in the shower for 20 to 40 minutes. 2 cups Epsom salts, 1 cup baking soda, and ten drops of lavender are much better. Make sure you're drinking enough water. Epsom salts, which are composed of magnesium and sulfate, can be added to a bath to help you relax and detox by flooding your cells with magnesium. Baking soda (sodium bicarbonate) aids detoxification and alkalinizes your body, while lavender oil relaxes your nervous system and lowers cortisol.

4. Before going to bed, take magnesium or melatonin.

Your body releases melatonin in the evening, making you drowsy, but it only does so if it receives the correct signals from your surroundings. Because melatonin is regarded as the "dark hormone," your body will not release it until the lights are turned off. Dim light should be switched on as soon as 8 or 9 p.m. Before going to bed, dim the lights to signal your brain that it's time to sleep. Ideally, you should obtain at least 8 hours of sleep each night. You should also aim to turn off the lights by 10: 30 p.m.

Chapter Twelve

ALCOHOL AND SOCIAL LIFE

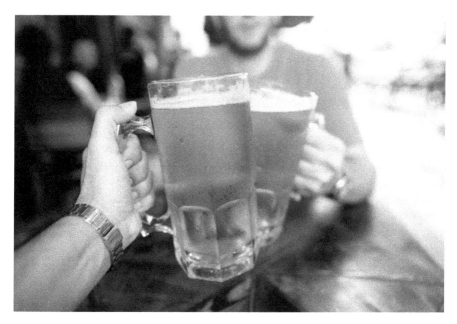

W hen you've tried to quit smoking, I've found that drinking alcohol and spending time with other smokers are two of the most common triggers for relapse. These instances can be your biggest downfalls in terms of relapses if you have a rubber arm that's easily twisted.

Inhibitions are lessened by alcohol.

One of the most serious issues with alcohol is that it weakens a person's inhibitions and resolve. Reduced inhibitions increase the chance of relapse when trying to quit smoking. After a few drinks, all of your willpower vanishes. Your lizard brain takes over and doesn't care about the past or the future, how difficult it was for you to overcome nicotine withdrawal or the implications of continuing to smoke.

To begin, I advise abstaining from alcohol. I understand that it appears to be a silly idea because you want to be able to drink without smoking. On the other hand, going alcohol-free will allow you to deal with the triggers that may develop in circumstances where others are drinking (without the added disadvantage of alcohol lowering your resolve).

You can think of it as a health kick, and I have to confess that going alcohol-free for the night while everyone else is getting drunk is both entertaining and eye-opening. Drink cranberry juice with Coke and lime or any other non-alcoholic beverage that appeals to you. Socialize as usual while paying attention to and working through any triggers that arise. It may not be pleasurable, but it is the first step toward overcoming your negative associations with smoking, alcohol, and social settings.

Make a plan for how you'll deal with the need to smoke when it arises. Go to the bathroom or go outside for a breath of fresh air. Allow your desire to smoke to wash over you and then feel it is released using the bring it on technique or imagine your inner self telling you to smoke.

Developing a New Routine

You are forming new healthy habits every time you successfully overcome your temptation to smoke in situations that were previously triggered for you. It takes time to form new habits, just as letting go of old ones. You'll soon be able to socialize with other smokers while enjoying a drink without being bothered.

Other Smokers

In my experience, smokers who have a smoking spouse, coworker, or buddy have the highest relapse rate. It's far more difficult to keep your determination when everyone around you is smoking. Smoking can be a fun way to socialize and engage with others. You are constantly exposed to smoking if you have a partner or family member who smokes. If your pals smoke, you will be exposed to it whenever you are with them.

If folks at work smoke, you're likely to be surrounded by smokers at least five days a week. So, how do you handle the potential for conflict when you quit smoking, but your partner, family, friends, and coworkers don't?

First and foremost, you must recognize that you may be on your own in your attempt to stop smoking. It may be stressful and upsetting to feel alone on this road, but you must accept the truth that just because you are quitting smoking, it does not mean that everyone else around you is quitting as well. Some people may try to persuade or even force you to restart smoking. You may inadvertently or even purposefully pressure those around you to do the same when you quit smoking. They may feel threatened or resentful of your decision to quit, and their response may be to make it more difficult for you to quit.

So be prepared for the loneliness you may feel, as well as the retaliation you may receive from smokers in your life. Prepare to dig deep and discover your own inner power to get you through this adventure.

When I make important decisions in my life and am fully committed to seeing them through, the perfect individuals appear to assist me in overcoming my challenges. Therefore, I recommend that you speak with the smokers in your life. Sit down with them and tell them you're quitting smoking, as well as why quitting is so essential to you. Request their help and ask that they be considerate if they want to smoke while you're around.

Make it obvious that you are not expecting them to leave because you are. If they are ready, you can invite them to quit with you. But be sure you don't have any preconceived notions about what they'll do. It's up to you to decide what your smoking boundaries are in the presence of people who are smoking. You are the one person over whom you have complete control.

You can beg people not to smoke in your presence, but you will eventually have to cope with people smoking in front of you. Of course, you can always leave a location where others are smoking if you want to.

If someone is smoking near you, make sure you have something else to focus on. For example, distract yourself with your phone, an app, a game, or a nice book. When I observe people smoking, I find that focusing on the negatives actually helps.

Focusing on how unpleasant smoking is, how horrible it smells, and how much time and money smoking wastes will help you feel like you weren't losing out. Thinking to yourself, "Thank God that's not me," can help you remember why you left in the first place. If you take smoke breaks with your coworkers, you could experience a different form of withdrawal than nicotine: friend withdrawal. If you work in an environment with a dedicated smoking place, you may have smoking pals with whom you spend your breaks.

I recommend avoiding the smoking area to make the process go more smoothly. This may cause significant FOMO (fear of missing out), but you can still see these folks at other times. Eventually, seeing other people smoke won't upset you; you'll just feel sad for them. Typically, the first month is the hardest, and hanging out with smokers is akin to a freshly sober heroin addict hanging out with other addicts. This isn't helpful.

Although the presence of other smokers, quitting smoking does not have to be tough, and it may even motivate others to do so. Take the chance to reveal to your friends and family that you're quitting and would appreciate their help. At the same time, be considerate of other smokers and give them the option to smoke if they so desire. For example, tell someone to go have a cigarette instead of telling them they shouldn't. Reverse psychology works successfully with most smokers since they are rebellious at heart.

You can quit smoking and be an inspiration to others, regardless of whether your family, friends, or coworkers smoke.

Chapter Thirteen

NICOTINE FAQs

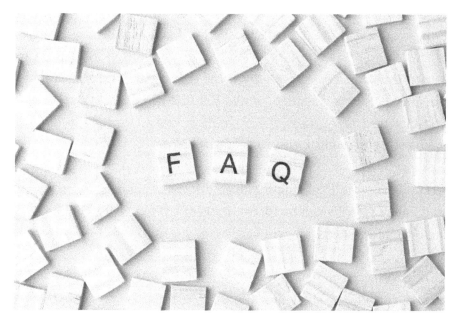

W## ill lowering the nicotine content of cigarettes make it easier for smokers to quit?

The FDA is looking at whether cigarettes could be made "nonaddictive" and whether or not the lack of nicotine would promote or deter individuals from smoking more.

Is it feasible to develop a nicotine cigarette that is not addictive?

That is the question that the United States is debating. With a new endeavor to examine the potential of a "low-nicotine" cigarette, the Food and Drug Administration (FDA) intends to respond.

According to the Centers for Disease Control and Prevention (CDC), more than 36 million adults in the United States smoke cigarettes, even though smoking rates have continued to decline.

Every year, 480,000 deaths in the United States are attributable to smoking-related causes, accounting for around one-fifth of all deaths.

In a statement, FDA Commissioner Dr. Scott Gottlieb said, "The overwhelming proportion of death and disease linked to tobacco is caused by addiction to cigarettes – the only legal consumer product that, when used as intended, would kill half of all long-term users." "Unless we alter course, 5.6 million young people will die prematurely from cigarette usage later in life."

According to the FDA, approximately 90% of adult smokers began smoking before the age of 18. So, in theory, if cigarettes contain less nicotine, fewer teenagers will become addicted.

Low-nicotine cigarettes may also aid die-hard smokers in weaning themselves off their daily nicotine habit.

So far, FDA authorities are only looking into the possibility and starting a public discussion about "nonaddictive" cigarettes.

In addition, FDA authorities are looking into expanding access to therapeutic nicotine products to aid people in quitting smoking.

They also announced that new restrictions for combustible tobacco products such as cigars and hookah, as well as electronic cigarette devices, will be delayed until 2021 and 2022, respectively.

Possible benefits and drawbacks

The American Cancer Society Cancer Action Network's policy principle, Katie McMahon, expressed optimism that this campaign will influence smoking rates.

McMahon told Healthline, "We are enthused about the idea of addressing nicotine and cigarettes."

She did, however, warn out that the FDA will need to work with experts and scientists to ensure that low-nicotine cigarettes do not encourage smokers to switch to other nicotine consumption methods.

"How does having different cigarettes on the market with different levels of nicotine affect the use of other products like e-cigarettes?" "McMahon stated. "It's impossible to reduce nicotine in cigarettes on its own."

According to Laurent Huber, executive director of Action on Smoking and Health, the program sounds like a "good way forward" if properly handled.

Huber told Healthline, "It clearly needs to be done well."

The oldest anti-tobacco organization in the United States is Action on Smoking and Health.

According to Huber, the FDA must be careful not to foster the growth of an illicit market for full-nicotine cigarettes imported from other nations.

Furthermore, individuals may mistakenly believe that these new "low-nicotine" cigarettes are safe to smoke.

Alternatively, rather than being completely weaned off nicotine, users may choose to acquire their nicotine fix through unregulated e-cigarettes.

Huber stated, "Nicotine addiction is not a benign disease." "We don't want to see an increase in nicotine usage among young people," said the group.

While Huber supports the FDA approach, he believes they should consider the risk that people will smoke more with low-nicotine cigarettes.

"You'd have addicted smokers looking for a nicotine high elsewhere," Huber added. "Some have wondered if people may strive to smoke or inhale more... to get as much cigarette smoke as possible in the hopes of receiving enough nicotine."

While low-nicotine cigarettes aren't expected to be available for months or perhaps years, Huber believes the U.S. government may take other actions to cut smoking rates.

Other countries' warning labels, he claims, are more graphic to prevent smokers.

Furthermore, some states continue to allow smoking in public areas indoors, thus increasing the risk of second-hand smoke.

How long does nicotine last in your body?

Nicotine is absorbed into your bloodstream when you smoke, chew tobacco, or inhale second-hand smoke from a cigarette.

The majority of the nicotine is then broken down into cotinine by enzymes in your liver. These compounds are eventually excreted in urine by your kidneys. Thus, the amount of cotinine you consume is proportional to how much nicotine you consume.

Nicotine's major breakdown component, cotinine, can be found in your body for up to three months after ingestion. The length of time nicotine lingers in your system is determined by how and how often you swallowed it.

How much nicotine will I consume if I smoke one cigarette?

Although the amount of nicotine in each cigarette varies, one cigarette is estimated to contain 12 milligrams (mg) of nicotine. This nicotine will be absorbed into your circulation at a rate of roughly 1 mg per minute.

Nicotine is measured in nanograms per milliliter (ng/mL) once it has entered your bloodstream. Cotinine levels in a nonsmoker's blood with no second-hand smoke exposure are less than 1 ng/mL. An average daily smoker's level is usually more than 10 ng/mL and can potentially reach 500 ng/mL. Between 30 and 50 ng/mL is the average.

Cotinine will normally be found in your urine for four days if you smoke infrequently. Cotinine can be detected for up to three weeks after you've been exposed to nicotine frequently.

The timing of your urine sample in relation to the last time you ingested nicotine determines whether or not you have a positive pee test. At 1,000ng/mL, the test may be positive if you are currently smoking; if you haven't smoked in over two weeks, a positive test could be over 30 ng/mL. Because each lab's positivity reference ranges vary, it's critical to discuss the results with your doctor.

How long will nicotine traces remain in your blood?

For one to three days, nicotine remains in your bloodstream, while cotinine stays in your bloodstream for up to ten days.

Nicotine in your blood can be identified using both qualitative (whether nicotine is present) and quantitative (how much nicotine is present) testing (how much nicotine is present). Nicotine, cotinine, and another breakdown product known as anabasine can all be detected using these tests.

Blood tests frequently provide false positives for nicotine. The presence of a chemical known as thiocyanate is mostly responsible for this. It can be present in foods such as broccoli and cabbage, as well as in several pharmaceuticals.

What is the duration of nicotine traces in your saliva and hair follicles?

It can take up to four days for nicotine and cotinine to be completely eliminated from your saliva.

Nicotine residues can be found in your hair follicles for up to three months after your last nicotine exposure. In addition, nicotine can be detected for up to a year after your last exposure, depending on the hair test performed.

Hair testing is an option, but it isn't as common as urine, saliva, or blood testing. This is because hair testing is often more expensive.

How can I know how much nicotine I have in my system? Are there any tests I can perform at home?

To check for nicotine in your system, you can use over-the-counter urine or saliva tests. These tests usually only give you a "yes" or "no" response, and they don't always tell you how much nicotine is in your system. Because doctors don't commonly prescribe these items, their accuracy and dependability are unknown compared to tests conducted in an employment office or a doctor's office.

<u>What factors affect the length of time nicotine remains in your system?</u>

While there are some broad criteria for how long nicotine stays in your system, it differs from person to person. Nicotine may leave your system sooner or perhaps linger longer, depending on your personal circumstances.

- How often you smoke
- People who smoke can be classified into one of three categories:
- Smokers who only smoke once a week are considered light users.
- Moderate smokers, or those who smoke three times a week or less
- Heavy smokers, or those who smoke on a regular or weekly basis.
- Nicotine residues are usually removed from your system within two to three days if you're a light smoker.
- Nicotine residues may be detected for up to a year after your last exposure if you're a heavy user.
- Your genetic makeup and your way of life

The length of time it takes your body to digest nicotine and drains it out is influenced by several factors.

These are some of them:

- The longer it takes your body to remove this toxin, the older you are.

- Genes: According to some research, Caucasians and Hispanics may metabolize nicotine more quickly than Asian-Americans and African-Americans.

- Hormones: Sex hormones are also known to play a role. Women may metabolize nicotine more quickly than men, especially if they are pregnant or on estrogen.

- Depending on their liver enzymes, different persons may metabolize nicotine at various rates.

- Medications you're currently taking

- The rate at which your body metabolizes nicotine might be affected by some drugs.

Medications that help to speed up nicotine metabolism include:

- Rifampin
- phenobarbital
- Medications that slow nicotine metabolism include:
- ketoconazole
- Amlodipine

How can you get nicotine out of your system?

Abstaining from all tobacco products is the most effective strategy to eliminate nicotine from your system. This allows your body's cells to concentrate on breaking down and excreting nicotine.

You can speed up the procedure by doing the following:

Drink more water: When you drink more water, your body releases more nicotine through your urine.

Exercise boosts your body's metabolism, allowing you to burn nicotine more quickly. Exercise-induced sweat carries nicotine and its metabolites with it.

Consume antioxidant-rich foods: Antioxidants can aid in accelerating your body's metabolism. Oranges and carrots are good choices. These meals also contain substances that aid in the elimination of toxins, such as fiber.

<u>Are there any negative consequences as the nicotine leaves your system?</u>

Cigarettes contain nicotine, which is the most addictive component.

Like coffee or cocaine, Nicotine can act as a stimulant in tiny doses. Nicotine becomes a relaxant when consumed in big amounts. It has the potential to reduce tension and anxiety.

Withdrawal symptoms can be triggered by ingesting lesser amounts of nicotine or completely refraining.

These are some of them:

- a strong desire to smoke
- increased hunger
- fatigue
- inability to concentrate
- headache
- constipation

- nausea

- diarrhea

- irritability

- anxiety

- depression

- insomnia

Your symptoms may be the most severe in the first few hours after you've quit smoking. These symptoms normally go away during the first three days of not smoking.

The severity of your symptoms and how long they last are determined by several factors, including:

- how long have you been a smoker

- what kind of tobacco products you smoked

- how much you smoke daily

Nicotine replacement treatments (NRTs), such as the nicotine patch, can help alleviate withdrawal symptoms as you gradually reduce your nicotine intake.

According to ResearchTrusted Source, utilizing an NRT boosts your chances of quitting Smoking entirely by 50 to 70%. If you use an NRT, you'll still have measurable nicotine levels in your body until you stop using it completely.

Last but not least

Nicotine traces can be discovered in your hair, blood, urine, and saliva if you smoke. It can be found in your saliva for up to four days after your last cigarette, and it can be found in your hair for up to a year.

Quitting using tobacco products is the most effective technique to eliminate nicotine from your body. Following are some things you can take to help speed up the process:

- drinking water
- exercising
- consuming antioxidant-rich foods such as oranges

CONCLUSION

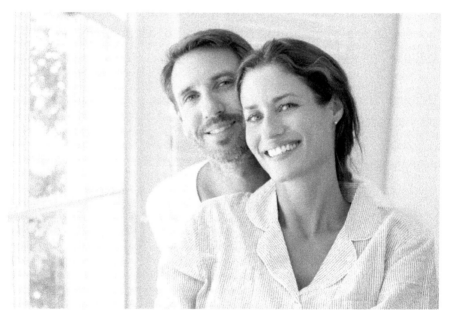

M any incorrect ideas, justifications, and maladaptive actions are based on nicotine addiction. Nicotine addicts frequently assume that cigarettes are required to function in everyday life. It's true that when you're addicted to a chemical like nicotine, you'll need more and more of it to avoid the withdrawal symptoms that begin the moment you put down a cigarette. However, it is also true that the cycle can be broken.

It's typical to believe that you need smokes throughout the day to help you get up, relax, digest food, or keep yourself occupied when you're bored, but you can live a healthy and happy life without them. It's vital to understand and overcome the incorrect cognitive patterns that excuse smoking when quitting. It takes patience and practice, but navigating the hurdles of early smoking cessation is possible.

The good news is that this period of quitting smoking is just temporary.

If you've read this book carefully, you've learned everything you need to know to turn your life around. Quitting smoking is not only about reducing your health risks but also about improving your relationships with others and ourselves.

Although it may seem hard now, follow this step-by-step program and you're sure to succeed.

It's up to you!

Lightning Source UK Ltd.
Milton Keynes UK
UKHW021841090223
416682UK00012B/713